Pediatric Gastroenterology and Nutrition

Christine M. Houser

Pediatric Gastroenterology and Nutrition

A Practically Painless Review

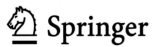 Springer

Christine M. Houser
Department of Emergency Medicine
Erasmus Medical Center
Rotterdam, The Netherlands

ISBN 978-1-4939-0448-8   ISBN 978-1-4939-0449-5 (eBook)
DOI 10.1007/978-1-4939-0449-5
Springer New York Heidelberg Dordrecht London

Library of Congress Control Number: 2014933121

Springer is part of Springer Science+Business Media (www.springer.com)

To my parents Martin and Cathy who made this journey possible, to Patrick who travels it with me, and to my wonderful children Tristan, Skyler, Isabelle, Castiel, and Sunderland who have patiently waited during its writing – and are also the most special of all possible reminders for why pediatric medicine is so important.

Important Notice

Medical knowledge and the accepted standards of care change frequently. Conflicts are also found regularly in the information provided by various recognized sources in the medical field. Every effort has been made to ensure that the information contained in this publication is as up to date and accurate as possible. However, the parties involved in the publication of this book and its component parts, including the author, the content reviewers, and the publisher, do not guarantee that the information provided is in every case complete, accurate, or representative of the entire body of knowledge for a topic. We recommend that all readers review the current academic medical literature for any decisions regarding patient care.

Preface

Keeping all of the relevant information at your fingertips in a field as broad as pediatrics is both an important task and quite a lot to manage. Add to that the busy schedule most physicians and physicians-to-be carry of a practice or medical studies, family life, and sundry other personal and professional obligations, and it can be daunting. Whether you would like to keep your knowledge base up to date for your practice, are preparing for the general pediatric board examination or recertification, or are just doing your best to be well prepared for a ward rotation, *Pediatric Gastroenterology and Nutrition* can be an invaluable asset.

This book brings together the information from several major pediatric board review study guides, and more review conferences than any one physician would ever have time to personally attend, so that you can review it at your own pace. It's important, especially if there isn't a lot of uninterrupted study time available, to find materials that make the study process as efficient and flexible as possible. What makes this book additionally unusual among medical study guides is its design using "bite-sized" chunks of information that can be quickly read and processed. Most information is presented in a question-and-answer (Q & A) format that improves attention and focus and ultimately learning. Critically important for most in medicine, it also enhances the speed with which the information can be learned.

Because the majority of information is in Q & A format, it is also much easier to use the information in a few minutes of downtime at the hospital or the office. You don't need to get deeply into the material to understand what you are reading. Each question and answer is brief – not paragraphs long as is often the case in medical review books – which means that the material can be moved through rapidly, keeping the focus on the most critical information.

At the same time, the items have been written to ensure that they contain the necessary information. Very often, information provided in review books raises as many questions as it answers. This interferes with the study process, because the learner either has to look up the additional information (time loss and hassle) or skip the information entirely – which means not really understanding and learning it. This book keeps answers self-contained, meaning that any needed information is provided either directly in the answer or immediately following it – all without lengthy text.

To provide additional study options, questions and answers are arranged in a simple two-column design, making it possible to easily cover one side and quiz yourself, or use the book for quizzing in pairs or study groups.

For a few especially challenging topics, or for the occasional topic that is better presented in a regular text style, a text section has been provided. These sections precede the larger Q & A section for that topic (so, for example, gastroenterology text sections will precede the Q & A section for gastroenterology). It is important to note that when text sections are present, they are not intended as an overview or an introduction to the Q & A section. They are stand-alone topics simply found to be more usefully presented as clearly written and relatively brief text sections.

The materials utilized in *Practically Painless Pediatrics* have been tested by residents and attendings preparing for the general pediatric board examination, or the recertification examination, to ensure that both the approach and content are on target. All content has also been reviewed by attending and specialist pediatricians to ensure its quality and understandability.

If you are using these materials to prepare for an exam, this can be a great opportunity to thoroughly review the many areas involved in pediatric practice and to consolidate and refresh the knowledge developed through the years so far. *Practically Painless Pediatrics* are available to cover the breadth of the topics included in the general pediatric board examination. It is important to note that, for some infectious disease topics also related to gastroenterology, additional materials can be found in the *Practically Painless Pediatrics* Infectious Disease book.

The formats and style in which materials are presented in *Practically Painless Pediatrics* utilize the knowledge gained about learning and memory processes over many years of research into cognitive processing. All of us involved in the process of creating it sincerely hope that you will find the study process a bit less onerous with this format and that it becomes at least at times an exciting adventure to refresh or build your knowledge.

Brief Guidance Regarding the Use of the Book

Items which appear in **bold** indicate topics known to be frequent board examination content. On occasion, an item's content is known to be very specific to previous board questions. In that case, the item will have "popular exam item" beneath it.

At times, you will encounter a Q & A item that covers the same content as a previous item. These items are worded differently and often require you to process the information in a somewhat different way, compared to the previous version. This variation in the way questions from particularly challenging or important content areas are asked is not an error or an oversight. It is simply a way to easily and automatically practice the information again. These occasional repeat items are designed to increase the probability that the reader will be able to retrieve the information when it is needed – regardless of how the vignette is presented on the exam or how the patient presents in a clinical setting.

Occasionally, a brand name for a medication or a piece of medical equipment is included in the materials. These are indicated with the trademark symbol (®) and are not meant to indicate an endorsement of, or recommendation to use, that brand name product. Brand names are occasionally included only to make processing of the study items easier, in cases in which the brand name is significantly more recognizable to most physicians than the generic name would be.

The specific word choice used in the text may at times seem informal to the reader and occasionally a bit irreverent. Please rest assured that no disrespect is intended to anyone or any discipline, in any case. The mnemonics or the comments provided are only intended to make the material more memorable. The informal wording is often easier to process than the rather complex or unusual wording many of us in the medical field have become accustomed to. That is why rather straightforward wording is sometimes used, even though it may at first seem unsophisticated.

Similarly, visual space is provided on the page, so that the material is not closely crowded together. This improves the ease of using the material for self- or group quizzing and minimizes time potentially wasted identifying which answers belong to which questions.

The reader is encouraged to use the extra space surrounding items to make notes or add comments for himself or herself. Further, the Q & A format is particularly well suited to marking difficult or important items for later review and quizzing. If you are utilizing the book for exam preparation, please consider making a system in advance to indicate which items you'd like to return to, which items have already been repeatedly reviewed, and which items do not require further review. This not only makes the study process more efficient and less frustrating, but it can also offer a handy way to know which items are most important for last-minute review – frequently a very difficult "triage" task as the examination time approaches.

Finally, consider switching back and forth between topics under review to improve processing of new items. Trying to learn and remember many information items on similar topics is often more difficult than breaking the information into chunks by periodically switching to a different topic.

Ultimately, the most important aspect of learning the material needed for board and ward examinations is what we as physicians can bring to our patients – and the amazing gift that patients entrust to us in letting us take an active part in their health. With that focus in mind, the task at hand is not substantially different from what each examination candidate has already done successfully in medical school and in patient care. Keeping that uppermost in our minds, board examination studying should be both a bit less anxiety provoking and a bit more palatable. Seize the opportunity, and happy studying to all!

Rotterdam, The Netherlands   Christine M. Houser

About the Author

Dr. Houser completed her medical degree at the Johns Hopkins University School of Medicine, after spending 4 years in graduate training and research in cognitive neuropsychology at George Washington University and the National Institutes of Health (NIH). Her Master of Philosophy degree work focused on the processes involved in learning and memory, and during this time she was a four-time recipient of training awards from the NIH. Dr. Houser's dual interests in cognition and medicine led her naturally toward teaching and "translational cognitive science" – finding ways to apply the many years of cognitive research findings about learning and memory to how physicians and physicians-in-training might more easily learn and recall the vast quantities of information required for medical studies and practice.

Content Reviewers

For Gastroenterology Topics

Ebony Beaudoin, M.D.
Assistant Professor, Department of Pediatrics
Division of Community and General Pediatrics
University of Texas – Houston Medical School
Houston, TX, USA

Emma Archibong Omoruyi, M.D., M.P.H.
Assistant Professor, Department of Pediatrics
Division of Community and General Pediatrics
University of Texas – Houston Medical School
Houston, TX, USA

Lisa de Ybarrondo, M.D.
Assistant Professor, Department of Pediatrics
Division of Community and General Pediatrics
University of Texas – Houston Medical School
Houston, TX, USA

For Nutrition Topics

Sigrid Bairdain, M.D., M.P.H.
Research Fellow, Department of Pediatric Surgery
Boston Children's Hospital
Boston, MA, USA

Kenya M. Parks, M.D.
Assistant Professor, Department of Pediatrics
Division of Community and General Pediatrics
University of Texas – Houston Medical School
Houston, TX, USA

Contents

1 The Bilirubin Pathway 1

2 Selected Gastroenterology Topics 5
Hirschsprung's Disease Pathophysiology 5
Carcinoid Tumors 6
Inflammatory Bowel Disease 7
    Crohn's disease 7
    Ulcerative colitis 9
Lactase Deficiency 11
    Lactase deficiency in pediatrics 11
    Lactase deficiency in adults 12
    Treating lactase deficiency 12
Menetrier's Disease 13
    What is it? 13
    How does it present? 13
    What happens in menetrier's? 13
    What will the histology show? 13
    Spontaneous resolution occurs in which patient groups? 14
    Is menetrier's associated with later development of cancer? 14
    Aside from menetrier's, what is the differential diagnosis
    for large gastric folds? 14
    How is menetrier's treated? 14
Veno-Occlusive Liver Disease 15
    Which vessels are damaged, and what is the problem? 15
    Which meds and toxins are the main contributors
    to this disease? 15
    How is this disorder diagnosed? 15
    How will it present? 16

How is veno-occlusive liver disease treated? 16
In addition to nodular regenerative hyperplasia,
what other related liver disorders are there? 16

3   General Gastroenterology Question and Answer Items 17

4   General Vitamin and Nutrition Question and Answer Items 133

Index 185

Chapter 1
The Bilirubin Pathway

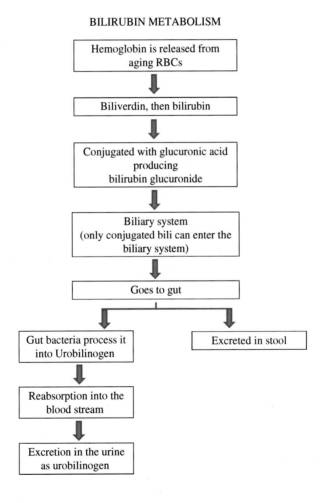

C.M. Houser, *Pediatric Gastroenterology and Nutrition: A Practically Painless Review*,
DOI 10.1007/978-1-4939-0449-5_1, © Springer Science+Business Media New York 2014

OBSTRUCTION
(liver able to conjugate, but not able to excrete)

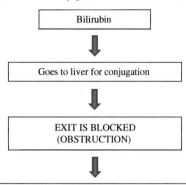

| Bilirubin |

| Goes to liver for conjugation |

| EXIT IS BLOCKED (OBSTRUCTION) |

| Then, it continues circulating as conjugated bilirubin (not protein bound because it is conjugated) |

| Urinary excretion as bilirubinuria (dark urine & light feces) |

HEPATIC DYSFUNCTION OR INSUFFICIENCY TO LOAD
(liver unable to conjugate, or unable to conjugate the amount
produced)

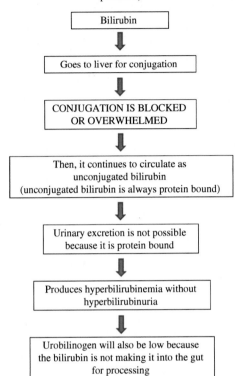

Chapter 2
Selected Gastroenterology Topics

Hirschsprung's Disease Pathophysiology

Hirschsprung's disease results from inadequate migration of neural crest cells from the proximal to the distal gut. If these cells don't make it to part of the gut, neither Meissner's nor Auerbach's plexi can form. These nerve plexi are needed to allow the gut to relax (among other functions).

Because the pathophysiology of the disorder is the failure of the migrating neural cells to get the whole way to the end of the digestive system, the anus is *always* affected. When we check for rectal/anal tone, it will always be normal because in a Hirschsprung's patient, **the gut is unable to relax without those plexi**.

The normal gut BEFORE the part lacking the plexi is the part that can dilate – and it does, eventually becoming overdistended, which can lead to enterocolitis and toxic megacolon.

Most patients present in the neonatal period, but some with only mild disease present later with constipation and failure to thrive, or even in adulthood with a history of chronic constipation without incontinence.

Only surgery can "correct" the problem in Hirschsprung's, and of course it is not a true correction of the problem. Surgery offers a mechanical way to prevent dangerous colon dilation and hopefully to allow the patient to be continent of stool.

This pathophysiology is different from severing the connection between the gut and the spinal nerves, as in spinal trauma, which results in *lax* rectal tone.

C.M. Houser, *Pediatric Gastroenterology and Nutrition: A Practically Painless Review*,
DOI 10.1007/978-1-4939-0449-5_2, © Springer Science+Business Media New York 2014

Carcinoid Tumors

Carcinoid tumors develop from neural crest cells that have migrated into the gastrointestinal and pulmonary systems where they live near the submucosa. These cells are called **enterochromaffin cells**.

Carcinoid tumors are **most typically found in the GI tract**, but they can occur anywhere that embryonic gut tissue went (including less well-known spots such as the thymus, gonads, kidney, and uterine cervix).

Carcinoid tumors is the most common tumor of the small bowel. It **most frequently occurs in the appendix** (41 %) and is the **most common appendiceal tumor** (frequently tested item).

Carcinoid tumor cells usually **produce small peptides and serotonin metabolites** that **are vasoactive**. This produces the classic clinical presentation of **carcinoid syndrome** – a patient complaining of periodic skin flushing, abdominal cramping, and diarrhea. Patients may also complain of wheezing, excessive salivation, or lacrimation. Occasionally heart valve fibrosis results from the actions of the peptides.

Many patients will not have any symptoms from these tumors, unless they produce an obstruction. Carcinoid tumor is frequently found incidentally while resecting for something else.

Histologically, enterochromaffin cells look like other neuroendocrine cells (they have a lot of cytoplasmic granules). Malignant cells cannot be differentiated from benign cells with the light microscope.

Carcinoid tumors progress through several stages in a predictable way. **First the tumor spreads locally** by tissue invasion. It **then** invades **local lymph nodes**. Finally, **metastases develop in distant organs**. The most favorite organ for carcinoid metastases is the liver. (Metastases in the liver are also especially likely to produce the symptoms described above. The area is very vascular, and the peptides produced are often dumped directly into the circulation, rather than being processed by the liver. If the liver has the opportunity to process the peptides it will usually inactivate them.) Metastases can also occur to many other tissues, such as retroperitoneal and supraclavicular lymph nodes, ovaries, skin, brain, or bone.

A **marker** for carcinoid tumor is available. It is 5-hydroxyindoleacetic acid (**5-HIAA**) which is a urinary metabolite resulting from the processing of serotonin. This is collected in a "**24-hour urine**." (A diagnostic that requires you to collect all of the urine produced by the patient over a 24-h period.)

Although some chemotherapy is available, **carcinoid tumors must be cut out**. Overall survival at 5 years is around 75 %, with substantially better survival for those patients who had only local disease.

Inflammatory Bowel Disease

Both Crohn's disease and ulcerative colitis (UC) clearly have both a genetic and an environmental component. Neither the genetics nor the environmental factors responsible have been identified yet. Crohn's disease has a 50 % concordance in monozygotic twins. Geography is a known risk factor, as individuals who emigrate from a low-risk area to a high-risk area improve their chances of developing these diseases.

Inflammatory bowel disease is the leading cause of gut inflammation in children older than 1 year in developed nations.

Both diseases are thought to result from a dysregulation of the inflammation normally present in the gut, as a response to the various pathogens and toxins it routinely encounters.

Crohn's Disease

Presentation

Around one-third of the individuals who will eventually develop Crohn's disease present in childhood or adolescence. Twice as many males develop the disease in childhood, as females. In adulthood, however, males and females are equally likely to develop the disease.

Course and complications

Recurrent bouts of abdominal pain, diarrhea, and rectal bleeding (small quantities) are the usual presentation. Patients tend to be especially tender in the right lower quadrant. (The diarrhea results from malabsorption and bacterial overgrowth.) Viral illnesses and gut bacterial infections often precede exacerbations. *C. difficile* infections are especially linked to flare-ups.

Patients with colonic disease have more extraintestinal (outside of the gut) manifestations of Crohn's disease and are usually harder to treat overall. (*Examples of extraintestinal conditions important in Crohn's are oral ulcers, erythema nodosum, arthritis, and digital clubbing.*)

Crohn's disease increases the patient's likelihood of dying by about 10 %, over the course of 20 years.

Abscesses, fistulas, strictures, and obstruction are common.

Perianal disease is very common.

Growth failure with a decrease in height velocity is common in children with Crohn's and may progress to short stature and pubertal delay.

Disease is most often present in the terminal ileum, although it can occur through the GI system.

Terminal ileal disease is associated with B12 deficiency.

Duodenal lesions sometimes lead to iron deficiency and anemia.

Patients are at increased risk for adenocarcinoma (though less so than UC patients).

There is evidence that there may be an increased risk of lymphoma in Crohn's patients.

Patients are at risk for associated autoimmune-related disorders such as ankylosing spondylitis, arthritis, and primary sclerosing cholangitis.

Work-Up

Colonoscopy with biopsy (depending on suspected location of lesions).

Upper endoscopy with biopsy (pathology should be of full thickness in some cases and feature granulomas, fissures, and skip lesions).

Barium upper GI with small bowel follow-through or magnetic resonance (MR) enterography (to avoid radiation exposure) for areas affected not accessible to endoscopy.

CT scanning useful to determine the extent of disease.

Video capsule endoscopy an option for small bowel inspection in patients >10 years.

Laboratory testing often demonstrates anemia, low protein, and high ESR or C-reactive protein. Normal studies do not exclude the diagnosis!

Treatment

Surgery is considered if medical therapy fails, but it is often not successful, because the disease is so diffusely present throughout the gut.

Medical therapy options are the following:

Bowel rest with parenteral nutrition.

Elemental diet may have some role in inducing remissions.

Sulfasalazine (sulfapyridine with 5-aminosalicylate) – used for prophylaxis (and sometimes for mild exacerbations). Good for lower (terminal ileum and colonic) disease only, because the medication does not become active until it is cleaved by bacteria in the colon. Sulfasalazine is given with *folate*, because sulfasalazine interferes with folate absorption.

A high dose is given in acute disease, but a somewhat lower dose may be used after resolution of the acute situation in an attempt to keep the patient in remission.

Note: **Rowasa, Pentasa, Asacol, sulfasalazine, mesalamine, and 5-ASA are all different versions of the same medication.** *Sulfasalazine has a sulfur moiety, while mesalamine does not. Mesalamine can be used for upper GI disease.*

Pentasa is effective for both upper and lower GI disease. A high dose is given for active disease and a moderate dose if it is used for prophylaxis/maintenance.

Rowasa is used with lower GI disease and comes in enema or suppository forms.

Antibiotics ciprofloxacin and metronidazole – These agents are helpful in decreasing inflammation and symptoms and are used with most exacerbations.

Prednisone is the first-line treatment, after sulfasalazine. The usual dose is 1–2 mg/kg/24 h to a maximum of 60 mg per dose, given once or twice per day, for 4–6 weeks. The dose is then tapered very slowly.

Hydrocortisone enemas are also sometimes utilized for mild disease limited to the colon.

Immunosuppressives azathioprine and 6-mercaptopurine – These agents are used when other agents have not been effective or sometimes in an attempt to decrease the amount of steroid the patient requires. They seem to decrease fistula formation as well as decrease disease manifestations overall. *Cyclosporine* has also been used in adults, but its appropriate use in children is not yet certain.

Infliximab, also known as anti-TNF-alpha antibody – Infusions every 2–3 months have been attempted to maintain remission. Its cost–benefit in this disorder is not yet clear.

Ulcerative Colitis

Presentation

Somewhat more common in males than females. The incidence of UC is holding steady, unlike the incidence of Crohn's, which has been increasing. UC is most commonly seen in individuals of North American and European ancestry. It is least common in those of Japanese and South African ancestry. About 20 % of patients with UC present under the age of 20 years.

UC also begins with abdominal or rectal pain, blood per rectum, and diarrhea – although sometimes patients may experience constipation in response to pain with defecation. Symptoms must last for more than 2–3 weeks to consider UC as a diagnosis. Growth failure and/or delayed puberty is a common presentation in children.

Use of NSAIDs and enteric infections may contribute to the onset of new exacerbations.

Course and complications

Typically begins at rectum and works its way proximally (limited to colon).

Disease limited to the rectum is typically more difficult to treat but has fewer systemic problems associated with it.

The more severe the disease is in its initial presentation, the more severe the course is likely to be.

The risk of colon cancer increases significantly after UC has been present for 10 years. If the UC is limited to the descending colon, only, then the cancer risk is lessened.

The extraintestinal complications most often seen with UC are the following:

Primary sclerosing cholangitis, chronic active hepatitis, ankylosing spondylitis, and pyoderma gangrenosum.

Work-Up

Barium enema is *not* usually helpful.

Endoscopy/colonoscopy with biopsy is preferred – although it should not be performed during an acute exacerbation, due to the risk of perforation or the development of toxic megacolon. Lesions should be diffuse, less than full wall thickness, and feature cryptitis and crypt abscesses.

In older patients who have had the disease longer, pseudopolyps, regenerating mucosa with atrophic surrounding tissue around it, may be seen.

When 10 years have elapsed since the diagnosis, colonic biopsy is recommended every 1–2 years to look for dysplasia. If dysplasia is present, colectomy is recommended. It is not clear from the studies available, however, whether this approach overestimates or underestimates the number of colons that should actually be removed.

Laboratory testing is nonspecific, often with anemia, low protein, and high ESR or C-reactive protein. Children with UC will have normal lab work more often than children with Crohn's do.

Stool should be checked for enteric pathogens, but even if they are found, IBD cannot be ruled out!

Treatment

20–30 % improve spontaneously in any given exacerbation.

Elemental feedings have not been found to be helpful in UC.

TPN is not helpful in the treatment of the disorder but is sometimes used to maintain the patient's nutritional status if surgery is a possibility.

The *5-ASA compounds* are used for mild disease, as are metronidazole and cipro (and sometimes clindamycin). The 5-ASA compounds sometimes take several weeks to have a significant effect. The usual dose for sulfasalazine is 50–75 mg/kg/24 h divided into two to four daily doses. The dose should start low and work up to avoid side effects (nausea, abdominal pain, headache). Ten to 20 % of patients will be allergic to sulfasalazine. These patients should tolerate mesalamine – the same compound without the sulfur moiety.

Moderate-to-severe exacerbations (and mild exacerbations with poor response to 5-ASA) are treated with *oral prednisone* 1–2 mg/kg/24 h given once or twice per day (with a 60 mg maximum per dose). In pediatrics, the patient cannot remain on this regimen for more than 3 months, maximum, due to the side effects.

If adequate response is still not obtained, or if the exacerbations are very frequent:

Surgery is an option.

Alternatively, *azathioprine, 6-mercaptopurine, or anti-TNF-alpha infusions* may be tried.

Proctitis – enema preparations of 5-ASA and hydrocortisone may be used.

Lactase Deficiency

Lactase deficiency in pediatrics

Congenital absence of lactase does occur, but it is rare.

Lactase deficiency is common in premature infants, because significant production of lactase does not begin until 34 weeks of gestation.

Lactase deficiency is seen after various infections affecting the brush border of the intestines, where lactase is produced. As the brush border returns to normal, the production of lactase does, too.

Lactase Deficiency in Adults

Lactase levels decline for most people beginning in late childhood. This decline continues into adulthood. Some ethnic groups are more likely than others to eventually develop lactase levels so low that digestion of lactose is a problem.

Interestingly, though, the correlation between the symptoms that the patient believes are related to lactose malabsorption and the actual amount of lactose malabsorption is not high. Gastroenterology texts recommend collecting a lactose hydrogen breath test for these patients, and correlating the results of that test with the symptoms the patient was experiencing at the time, if you want to determine whether the patient's symptoms are actually caused by lactose malabsorption.

Additionally, the severity of symptoms is *not related* to the quantity of lactose ingested. Also, many individuals with very low levels of lactase do not have symptoms.

Other causes of the symptoms patients often attribute to lactose malabsorption are fat malabsorption, incomplete absorption of other carbohydrates (which is normal), or intolerance of milk proteins.

Ethnic groups most likely to be affected by lactase deficiency:

Thai, Chinese, Korean, Indonesian, Native Americans, Australian Aboriginal Peoples, Arabs, Jews, Southern Italians, and certain African groups. (~15 % of white adults, 40 % of Asian adults, and 85 % of black adults in the United States.)

Ethnic groups least likely to be affected by lactase deficiency:

North Europeans, many African groups, and Indians.

Treating Lactase Deficiency

Slowing transit time helps (more time for the enzymes available to work) – whole milk and chocolate milk are both processed more slowly.

Hard cheeses have a lesser amount of lactose than soft ones.

Commercial preparations of lactase, to be consumed before meals, are available.

Yogurt is usually well tolerated because live culture yogurt produces its own lactase enzymes. Otherwise, patients who are bothered by milk products should avoid them, and be sure that they are getting adequate calcium.

Menetrier's Disease

What is it?

Menetrier's disease is a rare type of hyperplastic gastropathy. Menetrier's disease and Zollinger–Ellison both cause hyperplastic gastropathy.

Menetrier's disease has two forms, regular Menetrier's and a variation called "hyperplastic, hypersecretory gastropathy."

How does it present?

Protein-losing gastropathy (sometimes not seen in the variant version)

Hypochlorhydria (regular Menetrier's)

Normal or high acid secretion (hyperplastic, hypersecretory gastropathy)

Large gastric folds that affect the whole body of the stomach – antrum is spared

Weight loss

Vomiting

Epigastric pain

Anorexia

Hematemesis

Occult blood

What happens in Menetrier's?

CMV, or other triggers such as HSV, *H. pylori*, or *Giardia*, causes inflammation and histological changes. TGF-α is thought to be an important part of the disorder, but its role is not yet clear.

What will the histology show?

A full-thickness biopsy is needed to evaluate hyperplastic gastropathies.
Regular Menetrier's:

"Foveolar" cell hyperplasia with cystic dilation. Edema and inflammation. Decreased chief and parietal cells. Lost cells are sometimes replaced with extra mucous glands.

Hyperplastic, hypersecretory variation:

Parietal and chief cell hyperplasia

Spontaneous resolution occurs in which patient groups?

Children and postpartum women

Is Menetrier's associated with later development of cancer?

A matter of debate in the literature. Some series show that 15 % of affected adults develop GI cancers, but it is not clear whether the Menetrier's is a significant factor in *causing* the cancer.

Aside from Menetrier's, what is the differential diagnosis for large gastric folds?

Neoplasm (carcinoma or lymphoma)

Granulomatous disease affecting the stomach

Gastric varices

Infectious gastritis (CMV or *H. pylori*)

Eosinophilic gastritis

Zollinger–Ellison

Crohn's disease

How is Menetrier's treated?

Treat *H. pylori* if present – eliminating it sometimes eliminates the problem.

H2 blockers and other acid blockers are used, along with anticholinergics. The use of these medications may decrease protein losses through the effects on gut epithelial cells.

Occasionally, it has been treated with steroids, octreotide, antifibrinolytics, and monoclonal antibodies against the EGF receptor (epidermal growth factor receptor).

In rare cases, partial or total gastric resection can be used as a last resort.

Veno-Occlusive Liver Disease

Veno-occlusive liver disease is an uncommon form of liver disease *usually caused by medications or other toxins*. Although the patient develops symptoms of portal vascular obstruction, the large vessels are patent, and no clots are present in any of the hepatic vessels. The evolution of veno-occlusive liver disease can be quite acute, or it may develop over weeks to months.

Which vessels are damaged, and what is the problem?

The smallest venous vessels of the liver are affected (venules and very small veins).

The walls of these tiny vessels swell, then develop actual tissue thickening, and then sometimes fragment. Some nearby hepatocytes are often injured, as well.

Which meds and toxins are the main contributors to this disease?

All of the substances identified as causes are strong alkylating agents. In general, the larger the dose the patient was exposed to, the worse the damage. Anticancer regimens have a roughly 1 % likelihood (overall) of causing this disorder. Bone marrow transplant regimens, though, have been recorded to cause this problem in up to 54 % of patients treated (depending on regimen – fortunately it is not always so high).

These substances are also present in certain teas and folk remedies, such as "Jamaican bush teas" and comfrey.

Patients usually don't develop the disorder until 2–10 weeks after the start of the medication.

How is this disorder diagnosed?

This disorder is usually diagnosed by clinical presentation. Biopsy confirmation is not generally attempted due to the coagulopathy the disorder usually causes.

How will it present?

The acute presentation usually involves new onset of ascites and tender hepatos-plenomegaly.

The more common subacute presentation involves abdominal pain and hepatomegaly. Most patients later develop liver failure, jaundice, ascites, and coagulopathy.

Prognosis is poor, unless the presentation is quite mild (in which case the patient may actually have another disorder). Some patients go on to develop "nodular regenerative hyperplasia," a proliferative liver disorder, in which the veins are obliterated and disordered regenerative growth produces portal hypertension. (Nodular regenerative hyperplasia is more common in patients with myeloproliferative and immunological disorders.)

How is veno-occlusive liver disease treated?

Supportive care

In addition to nodular regenerative hyperplasia, what other related liver disorders are there?

"Noncirrhotic portal hypertension" is the descriptive term for portal hypertension in a liver that does not have cirrhosis. This can develop from veno-occlusive disease, but is also caused by distortion of nonvascular cells in the liver. Most commonly, fibrosis develops in perisinusoidal areas.

Toxins known to cause noncirrhotic portal hypertension include vitamin A, azathio-prine, methotrexate, arsenic, and vinyl chloride.

Chapter 3
General Gastroenterology Question and Answer Items

Is lactose intolerance common among infants?	No – It is seen in toddlers & children, though
What are the main symptoms of lactose intolerance?	Abdominal pain Bloating Flatulence Diarrhea
Milk protein allergy comes in two varieties. What are they?	IgE mediated & Non-IgE mediated
If a child has a problem with milk allergy and develops vomiting, diarrhea, eczema, and wheezing, which sort of milk allergy is it?	IgE mediated
Milk protein allergy that presents with enterocolitis, including hematochezia, anemia, and growth failure, is which sort of milk protein allergy?	Non-IgE
Elemental formulas are most useful for children with malabsorption problems & _____?	Severe milk protein allergy

C.M. Houser, *Pediatric Gastroenterology and Nutrition: A Practically Painless Review*,
DOI 10.1007/978-1-4939-0449-5_3, © Springer Science+Business Media New York 2014

If a child suffers from lactose intolerance due to an acute gastroenteritis episode, what nutritional practice will help to improve the situation?

Early refeeding

Recurrent bouts of periumbilical pain, vomiting, diarrhea, fever, *headache*, and *low pulse rate* may be what confusing diagnosis?

Abdominal migraine

(aka abdominal epilepsy – no seizure involved)

Children with abdominal migraine are likely to have a family history of what disorder?

Regular migraine headaches

What is the natural course of abdominal migraine?

Usually outgrown by adolescence

True "abdominal epilepsy" differs from abdominal migraine in what two significant, clinical, ways?

1. Altered level of consciousness

2. Shorter duration (minutes instead of hours)

How long does an episode of abdominal migraine usually last?

<6 h

What medications are helpful in the prevention of abdominal migraine (if episodes are very frequent)?

SSRIs
β-blockers
Tricyclic antidepressants

What medications are useful in the treatment of an acute episode of abdominal migraine?

The same ones used for regular migraine

(NSAIDs, ergotamines, antihistamines, etc.)

What is an appropriate work-up for a patient with known abdominal migraines who presents with abdominal pain?

Generally, the work-up is the same as for any other patient

(it's a diagnosis of exclusion)

What is the nature of the problem in α-1-antitrypsin deficiency?

Elastase, a connective tissue digester, is not properly inhibited

Which organs are primarily affected in α-1-antitrypsin deficiency?

Liver & lung

How is α-1-antitrypsin deficiency inherited?

Recessive

(Extra credit: Chromosome 14!)

In which ethnic group is α-1-antitrypsin deficiency most often seen?

North European ancestry (very unusual in those of Asian or African ancestry)

Is α-1-antitrypsin deficiency a common genetic cause of liver problems in kids?

Yes – it is the most common genetic cause

Many alleles on chromosome 14 are involved in α-1-antitrypsin deficiency (about 75). What is the name of the most severe form?

"ZZ"

Mnemonic:
Think of the lead singer for "ZZ" Top, living a hard life of smokin' & drinkin' on the road. This could do some severe damage to his liver and lungs

What is the name of the "worst" allele you could have for α-1-antitrypsin deficiency?

Z –
ZZ is homozygous, so it's the worst possible genotype

If an α-1-antitrypsin deficiency patient presents in infancy, how do they present?

Neonatal jaundice & hepatitis and sometimes acholic stools

In addition to jaundice, what else might be noted in the physical exam of an infant or a child with α-1-antitrypsin deficiency?

Hepatosplenomegaly

Is it common for α-1-antitrypsin deficiency patients to have asymptomatic intervals?

Yes

What lab abnormality is often noted during the early infancy of α-1-antitrypsin deficiency patients – even before they are diagnosed?

Persistent bilirubin elevation

(due to cirrhosis/cholestasis)

If an infant has cholestasis due to α-1-antitrypsin deficiency, can he or she become asymptomatic later?

**Yes –
often**

If α-1-antitrypsin deficiency does not present until adolescence or adulthood, how does it present?

Cirrhosis & ascites, usually

What is the name of the "normal" antitrypsin allele?

"m"

What vascular system complication(s) should you be most concerned about in α-1-antitrypsin deficiency patients?

Portal hypertension with varix formation

(and impaired clotting due to liver dysfunction)

In severe cases, how is the liver dysfunction of α-1-antitrypsin deficiency managed?

Liver transplant

What proportion of children with α-1-antitrypsin deficiency requires liver transplantation?

About ¼

Is it possible for a patient with α-1-antitrypsin deficiency to develop normal liver function over time?

Yes – ¼ will

What medication is sometimes used to manage the cholestasis that goes with α-1-antitrypsin deficiency?

Ursodeoxycholic acid

(aka Actagol®)

How common is perforation of the appendix in pediatric appendicitis?

Very common – 2/3 to 3/4 of cases

(the youngest children have the highest perf rates)

What age group is *most likely* to develop appendicitis?

Adolescents/young adults

Classically, what should you see on CBC and vital signs in an appendicitis patient?

CBC – mild left shift VS – low-grade fever

Classically, how should the patient describe the pain of appendicitis?
(3 things)

- **Gradual onset**
- **Poorly localized**
- **Migrating from umbilicus to right lower quadrant**

What is the eponymic name for the spot in the right lower quadrant where appendicitis pain often localizes?

McBurney's point

Why should you perform a rectal exam on a patient suspected to have appendicitis?

Both *appendiceal abscesses* and *retrocecal appendix* may be palpable/tender on rectal exam

(also rules out some other GI issues)

Classically, will the appendicitis patient be interested in food?

No

(may or may not have nausea & vomiting)

If a patient suspected to have appendicitis suddenly has relief of pain, what should you suspect?

He or she just perf'ed

(early perforation often has less pain – their condition will worsen in time, though)

How will the activity of a patient with appendicitis be described?

Lying still in bed

(should wince if you bump the bed)

Appendicitis patients usually have decreased bowel sounds due to inflammatory ileus. Why might they have diarrhea?

Irritation from a retrocecal appendicitis on the colon

What radiological investigations are usually performed to confirm appendicitis?

US or CT

(depends on the institution – US is more popular in pediatrics, but accuracy is operator dependent)

**How does appendicitis develop?
(3 steps)**

1. **Blockage (or rarely torsion) of appendix causes intraluminal pressure to increase**

2. **Increased pressure eventually decreases blood supply**

3. **Bacteria move in on the compromised tissue**

Does appendicitis run in families?

Yes

(no specific inheritance pattern identified, though)

Why does "ascites" occur?

Peritoneal fluid production exceeds absorption

What tissues are mainly involved in absorption of peritoneal fluid?
(3)

1. **Liver**
2. **Portal venous system**
3. **Lymphatics**

What blood abnormality can cause or contribute to ascites?

Hypoalbuminemia

(low albumin)

What are the two main complications to worry about in a patient with ascites?

1. **Spontaneous bacterial peritonitis**
2. **Respiratory compromise**

(with very large quantity of fluid, or very rapid increase in amount)

What is the minimal length of treatment for spontaneous bacterial peritonitis?

10 days

How can you tell that ascites fluid has a chylous (lymphatic) source?
(4)

1. Peritoneal fluid looks "creamy"
2. High fat content
3. High triglycerides (>400)
4. Few WBCs (despite creamy appearance)

Cirrhotic ascitic fluid is usually described as being what color?

Straw colored

More than 75 PMNs/mL of peritoneal fluid suggests that the ascites is due to what process?

Inflammation

(Infection has a much higher PMN count)

How is spontaneous bacterial peritonitis (SBP) treated?
(3 modalities)

1. **Antibiotics**
2. **Paracentesis**
3. **Correct the underlying problem**

Creamy ascitic fluid that is high in fat is most likely coming from what source?
(2)

Lymphatic obstruction or Trauma

(aka chylous ascites)

If a peritoneal tap contains blood or bile, what is the likely source for the ascitic fluid?

Trauma/rupture of a vessel or an organ

Why might a patient with a *single mediastinal tumor* develop ascites?

Compression of portal venous return to the heart

Or

Compression of lymphatic return (thoracic duct)

If the amylase value is high in the peritoneal fluid, what diagnosis should be considered?

Pancreatitis

If the glucose in the peritoneal fluid is *very low* (*<30*), what unusual diagnosis must be considered?

TB peritonitis

What do you need to order after obtaining peritoneal fluid for diagnostic purposes?

(6 categories)

1. WBC count & cytology
2. Gram stain & culture
3. LDH & pH
4. Amylase/lipase
5. Total protein & albumin
6. Cholesterol & triglycerides (TGs)

(look for infection, fat, & belly-related stuff)

What diagnoses must be considered in a neonate with ascites?
(3)

Lysosomal storage diseases
Cardiac abnormalities
Hepatitis (viral/neonatal)

(and other metabolic problems)

What dietary modifications help patients with ascites?

1. **Low salt intake**
2. **Water restriction**
   (75 % of maintenance)

Diuretics are sometimes used in the treatment of ascites. What complication do you need to be especially worried about in these patients?

Prerenal azotemia compromising the kidneys

(or possibly inducing hepatorenal syndrome)

What is hepatorenal syndrome?

Sudden loss of kidney function in a patient with liver disease

(mechanism unknown)

What is the name of the surgical procedure used to drain ascitic fluid to the venous system?

LeVeen shunt

(peritoneal venous shunt)

Why are LeVeen shunts currently unpopular?

High frequency of complications (especially infection & obstruction)

When would surgical portosystemic shunting be useful for an ascites patient?

If portal hypertension is a significant cause of the ascites

When should infected peritoneal fluid be reevaluated to determine the effectiveness of therapy?

48 h after antibiotics are started

How is peritoneal fluid evaluated for the effectiveness of antibiotic therapy?

Send for repeat culture

&

Repeat WBC count

In a patient with new-onset ascites, and no obvious etiology, what diagnosis (in general terms) must be ruled out?

Abdominal malignancy

If a patient with known, chronic, liver disease suddenly develops ascites, what "triggers" should you look for?
(3)

1. **Significant GI bleeding**

2. **Sepsis**

3. **New liver infection (causing acute liver decompensation, then ascites)**

What percentage of bezoar patients is female?

90 % (!)
(mainly trichobezoars)

Bezoars are most common in what age group?

Adolescents

(10–19 years)

Lactobezoars are most common in what patient group?

Low-birth-weight preemies

How are bezoars classified?

By their main "ingredient"

(hair, fungus, vegetable matter, etc.)

How do bezoars sometimes lead to pancreatitis and/or jaundice?

A "tail" sometimes extends through the pylorus, obstructing and irritating the biliary & pancreatic outflow areas

What physical exam findings suggest a trichobezoar?
(2)

1. Unusual balding pattern

2. Left upper quadrant mass (sometimes present with phytobezoars, also)

What psychiatric disorder is associated with trichobezoars?

Trichotillomania
Trichophagia

(patients obsessively pull out bits of hair, in this disorder)

What is a "phytobezoar?"

One made of plant matter

What gastric conditions make development of a phytobezoar more likely?

1. **Slow gastric emptying or dysmotility**

2. **Hypochlorhydria (low acid content)**

What dietary factors contribute to the development of lactobezoars?
(3)

1. Continuous tube feeding

2. Rapid feeding advancement in infants

3. High calorie density
   High casein
   High calcium/phosphate content

What gastric factor sometimes contributes to the development of lactobezoars?

Gastric dysmotility

How are trichobezoars usually managed?

Surgically
(often not amenable to endoscopic fragmentation)

How are lactobezoars usually managed?

Hold feeds for 48 h
Gentle gastric lavage

(*give IV fluids while you wait*)

What options are available for treating phytobezoars?

1. Meds (prokinetics, enzymes to digest it)
2. Endoscopic fragmentation
3. Surgical extraction
4. Acetylcysteine
5. Coca-cola

What common over-the-counter medications sometimes contribute to bezoar formation?	Antacids Vitamins & Psyllium (anti-constipation med)
What GI medications sometimes contribute to bezoar formation?	Sucralfate (coating agent) Enteric coated aspirin & Cimetidine (other acid blockers, too)
What is the most common cause of neonatal jaundice that requires surgery?	Biliary atresia
What *is* biliary atresia?	**A <u>progressive</u> disorder in which both intrahepatic, and some or all of the extrahepatic, ducts are obliterated (close off)**
What proportion of neonatal cholestasis cases are the result of biliary atresia?	About ¼
Is surgery to relieve outlet obstruction a definitive cure for the problems of biliary atresia?	**Generally, no – It progresses, and liver transplant is often required**
Which type of bilirubin is generally elevated in biliary atresia?	**Conjugated** (the liver processes the bili, but it can't get out!)
What surgical procedure is commonly performed for infants with biliary atresia when the *extrahepatic biliary tree is missing*?	The Kasai (hepatoportoenterostomy)
Why are biliary atresia patients sometimes so itchy?	**High-serum bile acids** (it may have to do with deposition of bile acids in the skin – mechanism is not really clear)

What is the most important determinant of long-term outcome for biliary atresia patients?

Age at surgery!

The younger, the better – even if the liver disease still progresses

What infection is especially likely in biliary atresia patients?

Ascending cholangitis
(very serious!)

What growth & nutrition issues are biliary atresia patients likely to have?
(2 main problems)

1. Fat-soluble vitamin deficiencies

2. Poor growth/failure to thrive (FTT)

What circumstances indicate that liver transplantation should be considered for a biliary atresia patient?
(4)

1. Liver failure (of course)

2. Intractable itching (aka pruritus)

3. FTT

4. Significant hemorrhage due to portal hypertension

If a biliary atresia patient develops raised yellow "spots" on the skin, what are the spots, and what caused them?

• **Xanthomas (fat deposits in the skin)**

• **Hyperlipid states often develop with liver dysfunction**

If a patient has pain typical of biliary problems, but no biliary abnormalities, what is the likely (biliary) cause?

"Biliary dyskinesia"

What are the two other common names for the pain syndrome of "biliary dyskinesia?"

1. **Post-cholecystectomy syndrome (if the patient already had surgery)**

2. **Sphincter of Oddi dysfunction**

Which gender is more likely to suffer from biliary dyskinesia?

Females

(as usual, with biliary issues)

In what age groups is biliary dyskinesia most common in pediatrics?

Late childhood & adolescence

Although it is not well understood, what is thought to be the problem in biliary dyskinesia?

Abnormal contractions

&

Possibly some functional (intermittent) obstruction near the sphincter of Oddi

What is the usual treatment for biliary dyskinesia?

Cholecystectomy

Or

Sphincterotomy

Will biliary dyskinesia patients have lab abnormalities? If so, what?

Sometimes –
Amylase & alkaline phosphatase may be high

How can biliary dyskinesia be managed medically (at least temporarily)?

Smooth muscle relaxants (nitro-based meds & calcium channel blockers)

What medications should be *avoided* in a biliary dyskinesia patient?

Narcotics (especially codeine)

(they could worsen sphincter of Oddi spasms)

What is breast <u>milk</u> jaundice?

Jaundice in an otherwise healthy infant – *aged 1–6 weeks*

How is breast <u>feeding</u> jaundice different from breast <u>milk</u> jaundice?

Jaundice in the third to fifth day of life in otherwise healthy infants is "breast feeding jaundice"

(assuming that the kid is breast fed, of course!)

What kind of hyperbilirubinemia is seen in either type of breast milk/ breast feeding jaundice?

Unconjugated!

What is the basic pathophysiology of breast *feeding* jaundice?

Dehydration

&

Inadequate calories

What is the basic pathophysiology of breast milk jaundice?

Abnormalities in the mother's breast milk (harmless, though)

When do you need to worry about kernicterus (bilirubin encephalo-pathy) in breast fed infants?

>40 mg/dL

What common birth trauma is known for causing transient hyperbilirubinemia?

Cephalohematoma

(as the blood is broken down in the hematoma, it briefly increases the bili)

When a neonate presents with jaundice, what life-threatening cause should you always consider?

Sepsis!!!

If an infant or its mother (during labor) received medications, what hyperbilirubinemia cause should you consider?

Medication side-effect

(sulfas, nitrofurantoin & oxytocin are common culprits)

What are the three main treatment options for breast feeding or breast milk jaundice?

1. **More frequent breast feeding**
2. **Formula supplements**
3. **Phototherapy**

What is "bilirubin rebound?"

When bilirubin increases rapidly within 24 h after *ending* phototherapy

When is exchange transfusion considered as a treatment for hyperbilirubinemia?

Level >30 mg/dL

Is sunlight effective as a phototherapy for hyperbilirubinemia?

Yes

(but watch out for sunburn!)

In pediatrics, where on the body is a cavernous transformation most commonly seen?

The portal or the splenic vein

What is cavernous transformation?

The development of collateral vessels around an obstructed vessel

In pediatrics, 50 % of portal vein obstructions are due to _____?

Idiopathic –
We just don't know

When a cause for portal vein obstruction can be identified in a pediatric patient, what is it likely to be?
(In general terms)

Structural abnormalities (vascular, biliary, or renal)

Although some patients with portal obstruction present very late – or not at all – how will symptomatic patients present?
(2 ways)

1. GI bleeding/hematemesis
2. Hepatosplenomegaly

Why might a portal vein obstruction patient acutely develop ascites?
(Liver function is normal)

Usually following a GI bleed – the RBC load sometimes causes a transient hepatic decompensation

Why might a portal vein obstruction patient develop steatorrhea or enteropathy?

Venous congestion can damage the mucosa

What activity modification might be needed for patients with portal vein obstruction?

**Splenic precautions –
If splenomegaly is present**

What are splenic precautions?

- **No contact sports (or must use a "spleen guard")**
- **No NSAIDs (risk of bleeding)**

When a celiac disease patient reaches adolescence, what beverage should be warned against?

Beer

(most are made from the offending grains)

Why is it important to give celiac disease patients a "trial of gluten" after their condition has normalized?

In some cases, gluten intolerance is transient

What grains contain gluten?

**Wheat
Barley
Rye &
Oats (to a lesser extent)**

What is the overwhelmingly common (80 %) presentation of celiac disease?
(4)

1. **FTT**
2. **Irritability**
3. **Explosive & foul-smelling stool**
4. **Vomiting**

At what age do celiac disease patients usually come to medical attention?

Toddlerhood

What are the main changes expected on evaluation of an intestinal biopsy in a celiac disease patient?	1. Villus flattening/atrophy 2. Lymphocytes in the lamina propria 3. Crypt hyperplasia
How common is celiac disease?	**Very common** **(1 in 300 counting asymptomatic individuals)**
In what part of the world is celiac disease most common?	**Europe**
What other diseases are associated with celiac disease?	Nearly all connective tissue/autoimmune disorders
What is the "classic" body habitus for a celiac disease patient?	**Short kid, bloated abdomen, & *wasted buttocks***
Although mucosal biopsy is the gold standard for diagnosing celiac disease, what lab test is nearly as good?	**Anti-tTG-IgA antibody test** **(A level 10× normal is expected in celiac)**
Why should you continue to consider celiac disease if the antibody test is negative?	**Some celiac disease patients are also IgA deficient**
Which possible celiac patients do *not* require biopsy confirmation?	Those with positive anti-TTG-IgA antibody tests + Celiac compatible HLA types (HLA-DQ2 or DQ8)
What hematologic abnormality is often found in celiac disease patients?	**Microcytic anemia**
How long should you expect to wait before a gluten-free diet improves a celiac disease patient to normal?	**Up to 6 months**
What oncologic diseases are celiac patients at increased risk for, if they do not stay on a gluten-free diet? (2 general sorts)	Intestinal lymphoma & Small bowel cancers (and sometimes other malignancies)

What two lab tests are more specific indicators of celiac disease than the previously used antigliadin antibody (AGA)?

AEA (anti-endomysial antibody)

&

Anti-tissue transglutaminase IgA

If children are found to have gall-stones, what are their usual complaints?

None –
Gall stones in kids are usually "clinically silent"

(may have right upper quadrant pain, nausea, and vomiting, if symptomatic)

Why do children on TPN have a higher likelihood of developing gallstones?

It is associated with decreased bile flow

What is the association to rapid weight loss and gallstones in adolescence?

Stones stimulate pancreatitis more often with rapid weight loss

Why would resection or poor function in the ileum contribute to gall stone formation?

Less functional ileum = less bile acids

(this means that the cholesterol is more concentrated & tends to form more stones)

What hematological disorder is famous for causing gall stones?

Sickle cell

(pigmented stones)

How reliable is Murphy's sign in children less than 10 years old?

(Murphy's = patient stops taking a breath in, when you push on the right upper quadrant)

Not reliable

(Their presentation is usually nonspecific)

When is ERCP indicated (mainly)?

For evaluation & possible treatment of common bile duct stones

ERCP = endoscopic retrograde cholangiopancreatography

For symptomatic patients, is medical therapy of cholesterol stones a good option?

No –
Low success rate *and they will recur when the med is stopped*

If a sickle cell patient is found to have gall stones, but is asymptomatic, what is the recommended management?

Cholecystectomy

(Gall stones have a high risk for complications in sickle cell patients)

What two common pediatric genetic disorders are associated with an increased risk of gall stone development?	Down syndrome & Cystic fibrosis
Colic is often attributed to GI problems. What is its actual etiology?	No one knows
What is different about the crying of a colicky baby?	There is a lot more of it – usually >3 h/day *(There is no difference in the quality of the cry)*
Colic usually "cures itself" by what age?	4 months
What are the two biggest dangers of colic?	**Child abuse (by worn-out parents/ care takers)** **&** **Overfeeding**
Both normal crying and colicky crying tend to occur most during what part of the day?	Evening
By definition, a colicky infant has what finding on physical exam?	**None –** **Well baby**
One of the main sources of colic is related to parental style. What is it?	Overstimulation (& difficulty reading baby's cues of fatigue)
What causes chronic active hepatitis?	**Many things** **(viruses, congenital disease, immunodeficiency, etc.)**
What are the three types of chronic active hepatitis?	1. Chronic persistent 2. Chronic aggressive 3. Chronic lobular
Which gender is more likely to develop chronic active hepatitis?	Females

How long should hepatitis persist to be considered "chronic active?"	**More than 6 months** *(no compromises – 6 months or it's not chronic active)*
If "bridging fibrosis" is part of the histological description of a chronic active hepatitis, is the hepatitis early or advanced?	Advanced
Scattered liver problems, with necrosis near the veins, are typical of what chronic hepatitis (associated with hepatitis B)?	Chronic lobular hepatitis
Spider angiomata & palmar erythema are buzzwords for what general problem?	**Chronic liver disease**
Which pediatric patients are most likely to develop sclerosing cholangitis?	**Those with inflammatory bowel disease**
Chronic active hepatitis is associated with what HLA types?	DR3 & DR4 (DR3 is worse)
Why are chronic hepatitis patients at risk for a life-threatening complication during commercial air travel?	Low cabin pressures may lead to varix rupture *(Oh, dear!)*
Are patients with autoimmune liver disease at high risk for recurrence if liver transplant is attempted?	**No** **(It does recur, but this is rare)**
What medication is the mainstay of treatment for chronic active hepatidites?	**Steroids** **(other immunosuppressives are also used)**
Why are chronic active hepatitis patients at risk for rickets and neuropathy?	Fat-soluble vitamin deficiency is common (vitamins D & E, especially)

What hand findings go with liver cirrhosis? **(3)**	1. **Palmar erythema** 2. **Clubbing** 3. **Dupuytren's contractures (tendons on palm of hand draw fingers in, decreasing hand function)**
Prominent veins on the anterior abdominal wall suggest what liver problem?	**Venous outflow obstruction**
Is congenital hepatic fibrosis a type of cirrhosis?	No – Cirrhosis requires fibronodular changes following hepatocyte death
What other organ is often abnormal in congenital hepatic fibrosis patients?	Kidneys
What liver abnormalities are seen in congenital hepatic fibrosis? (2)	1. Abnormal ducts persistent "duct plate" 2. Increased fibrosis (the lobular architecture is normal)
What are the main complications of congenital hepatic fibrosis? (3)	1. Portal hypertension 2. Hepatosplenomegaly 3. Cholangitis
What is the inheritance pattern for congenital hepatic fibrosis?	<u>Reces</u>sive (Fib<u>ro</u>sis has the same letter pattern as recessive)
Why might a congenital hepatic fibrosis patient have abnormalities on CBC?	Low platelets & leukopenia sometimes develop with hypersplenism
What is the typical LFT profile for a congenital hepatic fibrosis patient?	<u>Normal</u>
What commonly prescribed medications frequently lead to constipation in children?	**Calcium** **Opiates** **Antidepressants & other psych meds** **Mnemonic:** **Calcium, Opiates, Psych meds (COP) = COnstiPated kids**

How does the use of GI stimulants affect the prognosis for constipation?

It is bad –
More recurrences & failure to resolve

What is the usual mechanism of soiling by constipated children?

Rectum dilates, decreasing sphincter tone & sensation → stool leakage *around* the hard stool

Why do you need to perform a thorough back exam in a patient presenting with constipation?

A sacral dimple or tuft of hair suggests a possible spinal defect (causing constipation)

Why are stimulant laxatives bad as a long-term treatment for constipation?

Associated with nerve damage in the colon

At what age will most children require adult-sized enemas?

Age 12 years

How do dairy products affect constipation?

Increases constipation in most cases

What is caffeine's effect on childhood constipation?

Oddly, it increases constipation

Chronically constipated children with symptoms of an *acute abdomen* and a *palpable mass* should be ruled out for what emergency diagnosis?

Sigmoid volvulus

Why should you consider obtaining an abdominal X-ray series in a patient suspected to have constipation?

(3)

1. **Rule-out obstruction**
2. **Rule-out volvulus**
3. **To see how much stool is in the colon**
   (allows you to evaluate distention and helps to confirm diagnosis)

What portions of the GI system does Crohn's disease affect?
Which inflammatory bowel condition leads to "skip" lesions, fistulas, and adhesions?

Any! –
It prefers the terminal ileum & colon, though
Crohn's disease

What does a "skip" lesion mean?

The lesion in the gut is not continuous – there are normal areas between abnormal areas

How likely is a monozygotic twin to develop Crohn's disease, if the other twin has it?

50 % will also develop it

In children, which gender suffers from Crohn's disease more frequently?

Males

(In adulthood, it's equally common in males & females)

Perianal tags suggest which type of IBD may be present?

Crohn's

What proportion of Crohn's disease patients have perianal involvement?

¼ to ½

If a Crohn's disease patient primarily has terminal ileum involvement, what vitamin deficiency may develop?

B12

If a Crohn's disease patient primarily has duodenal involvement, what deficiency may develop?

Iron

What GI tumor are Crohn's disease patients at especially high risk to develop?

Adenocarcinoma

Why do Crohn's disease patients frequently develop diarrhea?

Malabsorption & bacterial overgrowth

What are the mainstays of treatment for Crohn's disease?
        (3 general categories)

1. **Immunosuppression**
2. **Anti-inflammatories**
3. **Antibiotics**

Which general types of anti-inflammatories are used to treat Crohn's disease?

Aspirin-based preparations

&

**Steroids
(both in local and systemic forms)**

Which types of immunosuppressives are usually used to treat Crohn's disease?

(3)

1. **Steroids**
2. **Azathioprine**
3. **Cyclosporin**

When should you consider surgery in the treatment of your Crohn's disease patients?

(5)

1. **Fistula**
2. **Obstruction**
3. **Abscess**
4. **Bleeding (not easily controlled)**
5. **Growth retardation**

The most-difficult-to-manage Crohn's disease occurs when which part of the gut is affected?

Colon

Why are Crohn's patients likely to develop renal stones?

(2 reasons)

• High rate of cell turnover increases urea → uric acid stones

• Can't absorb & break down oxalate well → oxalate stones

What is the definition of constipation-induced encopresis?

Overflow incontinence of stool around a mass of stool

What abnormality of rectal sensation do children with chronic constipation often have?

Reduced awareness of rectal distention

Does encopresis affect boys or girls more commonly?

Boys
(6:1)

Most cases of encopresis stem from functional chronic constipation. What other etiologies should you consider?

(3 general categories)

1. **Anatomic/mechanical problems**
2. **Metabolic**
3. **Neurological**

What is the difference between a food *allergy* and a food *intolerance*?

An allergy is the result of immune system factors –
Intolerance is due to missing enzymes, etc.

What is the link between food allergy and atopic dermatitis?

50 % of atopic dermatitis patients have a food allergy contributing to the atopic symptoms

What percentage of the pediatric population has a true food allergy?	About 2 %
Of the food allergies/reactions reported by patients or their families, what proportion can be confirmed with testing?	½
What percentage of infants with a food allergy will "outgrow" the allergy by age 3 years?	**40 %**
What are the most common food allergies? (5)	1. Eggs 2. Nuts 3. Milk 4. Wheat 5. Soy *(just think of what you most often see in your patients, and you will remember these)*
Cow's milk and soy protein allergy usually cause what type of allergic colitis?	Eosinophilic colitis (or eosinophilic gastroenteropathy)
Is cow's milk or soy protein allergy seen in exclusively breast fed infants?	Yes – Allergens may be transferred in breast milk
What are the signs that go with eosinophilic esophagitis? (3)	1. GE reflux (often with normal levels of acid production) 2. Dysphagia 3. Poor growth
How is eosinophilic esophagitis thought to develop?	Via food allergy (IgE or non-IgE)
Are other sorts of atopic disorders common in patients with eosinophilic esophagitis?	Yes
If a patient has an anaphylactic reaction to food, what medication must be prescribed?	**Epi-Pen!!!** *(prescribe for any patient with anaphylaxis to any substance!)*

How should the pediatrician manage a suspected food allergy (without anaphylactic reaction)?
(3 steps)

1. **Elimination diet (remove suspected food)**
2. **Reintroduce the food**
3. **Eliminate again to verify response**

If an elimination diet is not practical, or nutrition might be compromised by eliminating the suspect food, how else might you identify the food allergen?

Double-blind food challenges

How does "food poisoning" present?
(2 main markers)

1. **Fever, vomiting, & diarrhea 12–72 h after eating the bad food**
2. **Group outbreak**

What are the three ways that contaminated foods make us ill?

1. **Ingestion of preformed toxin**
2. **Toxin production in the gut**
3. **Direct mucosal invasion**

What food-borne pathogen is notorious for producing a carrier state – especially when antibiotic treatment is given?

Salmonella

(as in *Salmonella typhi* & "typhoid Mary")

When is antimicrobial therapy indicated for "food poisoning?"
(3 situations)

1. **Patients with poor immunity**
2. **Severe disease/bloody diarrhea**
3. **Patients with (chronic) GI comorbidities, such as IBD**

Is it possible to distinguish bacterial food poisoning from viral gastroenteritis, clinically?

(Most patients will tell you that it was definitely the food that made them ill)

No –
Unless the patient is toxic appearing (more likely bacterial)

How is gastritis defined?

Inflammation of stomach mucosa
(regardless of cause)

What is the relationship between gastritis and hemorrhage in children?

Most common cause of GI hemorrhage in school-aged kids

Patients in what sections of the hospital are most likely to develop gastritis/stress ulcers?
(2 settings)

ICU

&

Neuro ICU

(CNS disorders & CNS trauma predisposes to gastritis, especially)

What are the three main ways that infection with *H. pylori* is diagnosed?

1. **Upper endoscopy (with biopsy)**
2. **Urea breath test**
3. **Stool immunoassay**

Is dietary modification a useful strategy in the treatment of gastritis?

No

What is the mainstay of treatment for gastritis?
(2)

1. **H$_2$ blockers and antacids**
2. **Treatment of *H. pylori*, if it's present**

What is the "reservoir" for *H. pylori* infection?

Only humans!!!

What common complications occur in children treated with antacids?

Constipation

Or

Diarrhea

(change in appetite is also fairly common)

How is reflux different from vomiting?

It occurs without effort

How is pathological reflux different from physiological reflux?

Pathological is *greater in quantity and frequency* – and may cause complications

What age exhibits physiological gastroesophageal reflux most commonly?

Infants

(but it occurs in all age groups)

How do drugs & medications affect reflux?

Some decrease lower esophageal sphincter tone

What common drugs of abuse lower tone in the lower esophageal sphincter?
(2)

Nicotine

&

Narcotics

Which endocrine-related medications are known to decrease tone at the lower esophageal sphincter?
(3)

1. Estrogen
2. Prostaglandin
3. Somatostatin

What respiratory complications has reflux been linked to? (5)	1. *Reactive airway disease* 2. Pneumonia 3. Chronic cough 4. Stridor 5. Laryngitis
What very concerning complication must be ruled out when evaluating an infant with reflux?	**Near-miss SIDS** **(aka ALTE, an apparent life-threatening event)**
In young infants, the new development of pathologic reflux may indicate what non-GI diagnoses? (2)	Metabolic derangement & Infection/sepsis
When is surgery indicated for pathologic GE reflux? (2)	1. Mechanical problem 2. Medical therapy failed
What medical therapies are primarily used to treat GE reflux? **(2 general categories)**	**Prokinetic medications** **&** **Acid-reducing agents**
What is the first-line treatment for pathological GE reflux?	Diet modification (small, frequent feeds & thickening of formula)
What portions of the gut does Giardia infest?	**Duodenum & (proximal) jejunum**
How is Giardia spread? **(2)**	1. **Water** 2. **Fecal-oral direct spread**
Why might Giardia cause lactose intolerance?	Damage to the villi/brush border
What symptoms often develop *outside the GI system*, with Giardia infection? (2)	Urticaria & Arthralgia

What are the typical symptoms of giardiasis?	• **Watery, *foul-smelling* diarrhea** • **Abdominal cramps** • **Bloating** & *flatulence* *(perhaps we should say, "more foul smelling than average")*
In addition to acute giardiasis, Giardia sometimes produces another type of infection. What is it?	Chronic giardiasis
What medication is most commonly used for giardiasis?	**Metronidazole**
What is the most common GI complication of Henoch–Schönlein purpura (HSP)?	**Intussusception**
What is the basic mechanism for how HSP affects the GI system?	**It causes vasculitis** **(same as in the other systems)**
What types of vessels are affected by HSP's inflammation?	**Capillaries,** **Arterioles, &** **Venules** (most immune vasculitides affect small arteries only)
During what period of development does imperforate anus develop?	6–8 weeks of gestation
What proportion of infants with imperforate anus also has other abnormalities?	1/3
In general, imperforate anus is divided into two classes. How are these two classes distinguished?	By placement of the end of the gut above or below the levator muscle (referred to as "supralevator" or "translevator")
If a fistula exists to the GU system in a female with imperforate anus, where is it likely to connect to?	The vagina

If a fistula exists to the GU system in a male with imperforate anus, where is it likely to connect to?	The urethra (high imperforate anus)
	Or
	Scrotal raphe (low imperforate anus)
	(Raphe means the midline where the two halves come together)
Is it easier to achieve continence with a low-type or a high-type imperforate anus?	Low (90 %)
What is the most famous group of abnormalities with imperforate anus as part of the group?	**Vertebral anomalies** **Anus imperforate** **Cardiac anomalies** **Tracheo-** **Esophageal fistula** **Renal anomalies** **Limb anomalies**
Will infant patients with imperforate anus have an external anal sphincter formed at birth?	**Often, yes** (but no patent connection to the gut is present)
How is imperforate anus treated?	**Surgery** (High type requires a diverting colostomy, until pull-through can be used)
What part of the bowel is <u>always</u> involved in Hirschsprung's disease?	**The anus** **(varying lengths of proximal bowel are affected)**
What is the main problem in Hirschsprung's disease?	**Lack of GI nerve plexuses (aganglionic segment in the distal rectum)**
When do most Hirschsprung's patients present?	**Neonatal period (80 %)**
Are males or females more commonly affected with Hirschsprung's?	**Males (roughly 3:1)**

What is the most common cause of lower intestinal obstruction for neonates?

Hirschsprung's

What are the typical presentations of Hirschsprung's disease in the neonatal period?

Failure (or delay) in passage of meconium

&

Obstruction

As the infant gets older, Hirschsprung's can still present as obstruction, but two other possible GI presentations become more likely. What are they?

"Chronic constipation"

&

Enterocolitis
(less common)

(*Some will also present with FTT*)

What can be confusing about the enterocolitis presentation of Hirschsprung's?

Often includes diarrhea
(not what you think of with Hirschsprung's)

How does enterocolitis in Hirschsprung's disease usually present?

- Explosive, foul-smelling stools

- Fever (sepsis-like presentation)

- Bloody diarrhea

- Abdominal distention

What is the most common age for infants to develop enterocolitis with Hirschsprung's?

Less than a month old

Why might a Hirschsprung's patient be anemic?

Long-term blood loss in the large bowel due to chronic infections

What is the most concerning complication of Hirschsprung's disease?

**Enterocolitis –
It can easily produce sepsis**

On physical exam, what do you expect to find on rectal exam of a Hirschsprung's patient?
(2 options)

Good rectal tone & no stool

&

Sometimes explosive expulsion of gas and stool after digital rectal exam (squirt sign)

What is the most useful diagnostic to establish whether a patient has Hirschsprung's?	**Suction biopsy**
If an infant has not passed meconium at 48 h, should you automatically evaluate for Hirschsprung's?	**Yes** (suction biopsy)
If a suction biopsy is non-diagnostic, what other options do you have to resolve a possible Hirschsprung's diagnosis? <div align="center">(2)</div>	Full-thickness biopsy <div align="center">Or</div> Anorectal manometry (less accurate in neonates)
What is the other name for the type of enterocolitis that sometimes develops in Hirschsprung's disease?	**Toxic megacolon**
How does enterocolitis (toxic megacolon) develop?	**Intraluminal pressure in the colon thins the colonic wall <u>and</u> compromises its capillary blood flow**
In toxic megacolon (enterocolitis), what accounts for the severity of the patient's illness?	**Bacteria, toxins, & fecal breakdown products access the bloodstream**
How is Hirschsprung's treated?	**Colostomy/ileostomy until a pull-through is ready for use** *(laparoscopic & transanal procedures, as well as open, may be utilized)*
Ninety percent of inguinal hernias occur in which gender?	Boys
Inguinal hernias come in flavors: direct & indirect. Most pediatric inguinal hernias are which type?	**Indirect**
What does an "indirect" inguinal hernia mean?	**The abdominal contents are traveling <u>into</u> the inguinal canal** (through a potential space that was supposed to close up in development)

What is the name of the potential space the hernia (inguinal hernia) travels into?

Processus vaginalis

(it's supposed to close, but sometimes doesn't)

What is a "complete" inguinal hernia?

The contents make it to the scrotum or the labia

How is a direct inguinal hernia different from an indirect inguinal hernia?

Direct hernias "pop straight through" the inguinal wall, like a bank robber exploding a wall to get to the vault

(indirect hernias slide into an existing space or passageway to escape the abdomen, so they got out "indirectly")

In girls, what important organ may be found inside the contents of an inguinal hernia?

The ovary

Why would ascites or chronic lung disease increase a patient's probability of inguinal hernia?

Increased intraabdominal pressure

In children old enough to cooperate, what position should the patient be in when you examine for a hernia?

Standing

In what position should you try to reduce a hernia?

Lying down or Trendelenburg

(Trendelenburg means head lower than the body)

Pain in the groin with vomiting and abdominal distention suggests what serious diagnosis?

Incarcerated hernia

If you transilluminate a scrotal hernia, what do you expect to see?

The light should not come through

(hydroceles will allow the light to come through)

In addition to possible hernia, what other diagnoses should you consider in a child with acute groin or scrotal pain?

**Hip problem
(trauma, necrosis, infection)**

Or

Testicular problem (*torsion*, trauma, infection)

Should non-incarcerated hernias be urgently surgically corrected in infants?

Yes –
They have a high rate of incarceration in the first year

(not an *emergency*, but it is an *urgency*)

What is a Richter hernia?

One side of the bowel wall is stuck, the rest is free

Why is the presentation of a Richter hernia unusual?

Ischemic gut is possible *without obstruction*

An ovary herniated into the inguinal canal is often misdiagnosed as _____?

Inguinal lymphadenopathy

How is paralytic ileus treated?

(gut not moving well – usually in response to surgery or something else disturbing the gut)

Bowel rest alone is usually enough
(Supportive care, treat the underlying medical condition)

What general types of problems with the bowel <u>wall</u> can cause obstruction?
(4)

1. **Tumor**
2. **Stricture**
3. **Hematoma (most commonly duodenal)**
4. **Vascular or lymphatic mounds causing intussusception** (as seen in kids with Henoch–Schönlein purpura or Peutz–Jeghers)

Why is it a big problem if intestinal obstruction is not treated promptly?
(3)

1. **Risk of perforation**
2. **Patient comfort!!!**
3. **Possible bowel ischemia (depending on the mechanism)**

Mentally retarded children are at especially high risk for obstruction due to what problem?

Volvulus

(aerophagia, constipation, & sometimes medications affecting gut motility predispose them)

Abdominal pain due to obstruction usually has what characteristics?
(3)

- **Diffuse**
- **Moderate to severe**
- **Accompanied by nausea & vomiting**

What definitive management is usually required in cases of *pediatric* intestinal obstruction?

Surgery

(Adults usually develop obstruction due to adhesions – surgery is *often not indicated for them*)

What is the main diagnostic needed for patients with possible intestinal obstruction, and what are you looking for?

- **Flat & upright abdominal X-ray (abdominal series)**
- **Multiple air/fluid levels (± paucity of gas)**

Does a normal abdominal series rule out intestinal obstruction in kids?

No – up to 20 % may have normal films

What is the most common cause of intestinal obstruction in early childhood?

Intussusception
(*Specifically, between ages 5 months & 3 years*)

Why should you hospitalize a patient after a non-operative reduction of an intussusception?

**10 % will recur –
Usually in the first 24 h**

What is the key word to remember in describing intussusception?

"Telescoping"

(one section of bowel slides into a more distal part like a telescope)

Where will 90 % of intussusceptions be found?

Ileocolic area

Seventy-five percent of older children have a lead point that starts the intussusception. What proportion of children less than 2 years old will be found to have a lead point (with intussusception)?

Only 10 %

Which gender most often develops intussusception? What age range?

- **Boys**
- **5–10 months old** (various numbers are quoted in different sources – this is a good general idea of the main age range)

(seen, though, from 3 months to 6 years)

What proportion of intussusceptions can be reduced by contrast or air enema?

At least 2/3

(ileocolic intussusceptions, one of the most common sorts, are even more likely to be reduced)

When would you *avoid* using an air or a contrast enema in suspected intussusception?

If you suspect perforation or late diagnosis

If your patient has intussusception, what signs would make you think that he/she also has a perforation or is very late in the course?
(4)

- **Currant jelly stools**
- **Peritoneal irritation**
- **Shock**
- **Pneumatosis intestinalis** (air in the bowel wall) or abdominal air

What are the buzzwords for the description of abdominal pain with intussusception?
(2 classic descriptions)

Intermittent abdominal pain

&

"Draws legs up" during pain

Are currant jelly stools an early or a late sign of intussusception?

Late

(often not present)

What is the "classic triad" of an intussusception presentation?

- **Intermittent abdominal pain**
- **Vomiting**
- **Currant jelly stool (red & jellylike)**

What percentage of patients with intussusception will have a classic presentation?

20 %

Contrast enema reveals a "coiled spring" or "cervix-like mass." What is the disorder?

Intussusception

What physicians are involved in the non-operative reduction of an intussusception?

1. **Radiologist**

2. **Surgeon**
(due to 1 % risk of perforation)

What are the radiological buzz-words for intussusception?

"Coiled spring"

&

"Cervix-like mass"

How does an intussusception look on ultrasound?

A "tubular mass" or doughnut-shaped mass

(Doughnut shape if you view it from the end – Other typical descriptions are "bull's eye" & "coiled spring")

What toxic ingestion starts with GI symptoms and ends with GI scarring?

Iron

What is the explanation for the initial GI problems seen with iron ingestion?

Direct <u>corrosive</u> effect

(yikes!!!)

How do humans eliminate excess iron?

**Trick question –
We can't!**

(the gut regulates *absorption*)

How do *doctors* eliminate excess iron (from their patients, of course)?

Deferoxamine

(It's a chelator – allows renal excretion of the iron)

In addition to GI scarring, what other GI complications are seen with iron ingestions?
(4)

1. **GI bleed**
2. **GI perforation**
3. **Hepatic dysfunction (less prominent than with Tylenol®, though)**
4. **Acute bowel obstruction (due to scarring with healing)**

What radiological technique may be helpful in suspected iron ingestion?

**Abdominal X-ray –
Iron is radioopaque**

Why is it important to know the formulation of iron ingested?

It's the elemental iron that counts – preparations vary

We can lower iron levels in hemachromatosis with phlebotomy. Why wouldn't that be a good strategy with iron ingestion?

The patient is likely to develop shock

(He/she is often already GI bleeding)

How fast will patients develop GI symptoms after a toxic iron ingestion?

Less than 12 h

(GI symptoms are stage 1 of the iron toxicity stages)

If iron ingestion is suspected, but the patient does not present until GI symptoms are resolving, how should you interpret this?

Patient may be in stage 2 of toxic ingestion
Treatment is just as urgent!

(typically occurs about 6–24 h after the ingestion)

How common is irritable bowel syndrome?

Very common –
15–30 % of total US population

What is the underlying abnormality in patients with irritable bowel syndrome (IBS)?

Unknown –
Most studies have not found anything

Is there a genetic predisposition to IBS?

No

What symptom cluster defines IBS?
(4 symptoms)

1. **Recurrent abdominal pain & distention**
2. **Change in stool consistency (harder or looser)**
3. **Change in stool frequency (more or less often)**
4. **Relief with bowel movement**

How often must IBS symptoms be present to make the diagnosis?

At least 3 days per month

What is the first line of treatment for IBS patients?

Diet modification (usually high carb & moderately high fiber) & reassurance

How does lactose intolerance develop?
(2 ways)

Congenital
Or
Acquired
(usually through infection or chronic gut inflammation)

What causes lactose intolerance?

Lack of "lactase" enzyme

What are the typical symptoms of lactose intolerance?

Bloating, flatulence, pain, & diarrhea

If a patient has lactose intolerance, might he or she have blood in the stool or fat malabsorption?

No –
Signs like those tell you to look for another cause

What are the two main ways to test for lactose intolerance?

1. **Stool-reducing substances with pH measurement**

2. **Lactose breath hydrogen test**

What does a positive "stool-reducing substance" test mean?

Carbohydrates are present (they're not being absorbed – may have an enzyme deficiency)

If carbohydrates are not being absorbed in the gut, what happens to stool pH?

It will be low!

How does a hydrogen breath test suggest lactase deficiency?

Carbohydrates not absorbed by the gut are a source of H+ in the breath

Which ethnic groups are most likely to be lactose intolerant?
(4)

1. **Native Australians**
2. **Native Americans**
3. **Asian**
4. **African heritage**

How is lactose intolerance treated?

Avoid lactose

&

Give oral lactase supplements

What common childhood environmental toxin causes anorexia, intermittent abdominal pain, and sometimes vomiting or constipation?

Lead
(along with many CNS problems)

What is the most common congenital anomaly of the GI tract?

Meckel's diverticulum

(a yolk sac remnant)

Symptomatic Meckel's diverticuli are usually lined with what type of epithelium?

Gastric

(sometimes pancreatic)

Are males or females more likely to have *symptomatic* Meckel's diverticuli?

Males

(males & females are actually equally likely to have them, but males are more often symptomatic)

What is the peak age to present with a Meckel's diverticulum?	**2 years**
How large is a Meckel's diverticulum, on average?	**2 inches**
Where is a Meckel's diverticulum usually located?	**2 ft proximal to the ileocecal valve**
What are the two common presentations of Meckel's diverticulum?	**Rectal bleeding (painless)**
	&
	Obstruction
	(Meckel's are the most common lead point for intussusceptions resulting from a lead point)
In what situation is the bleeding from a Meckel's diverticulum likely to be more serious than average?	If the area bleeding erodes into the remnant of the <u>vitelline</u> artery
How is a symptomatic Meckel's diverticulum treated?	**Surgical removal**
What is a "Meckel's scan?"	**Technetium-99 scan – Gastric mucosa will take it up**
What is the most sensitive test for a Meckel's diverticulum?	**Meckel's radionuclide scan**
	(same as technetium-99)
If a Meckel's diverticulum is found incidentally, what should you do?	**Resection is recommended if:**
	Ectopic mucosa is present
	Or
	The bowel lumen is narrowed by it (increased risk of obstruction)
What is mesenteric adenitis?	**<u>Inflammation</u> of mesenteric lymph nodes**

In general terms, what usually causes (recognized) mesenteric adenitis?

Infection –
Both bacterial & viral, and not necessarily in the abdomen

What diagnosis is often confused with mesenteric adenitis?

Appendicitis

(the cecal or the ileocecal area is often affected by mesenteric adenitis)

What abdominal findings suggest mesenteric adenitis, on exam?

Patient cannot localize worst pain spot

Or

Point of maximum tenderness moves frequently

What infection is especially well known for causing mesenteric adenitis?

Strep throat

How can you differentiate mesenteric adenitis from other emergent causes of abdominal pain (with reasonable certainty)?

Abdominal ultrasound

Or

CT scan

How is mesenteric adenitis treated?

Supportive care

What serious complications are seen with mesenteric adenitis?
(3)

Intussusception,
Rupture,

&

Abscess formation
(rare, though)

In what organ systems will you see the effects of "milk allergy?"

1. **Skin (eczema)**
2. **GI (blood in stools, GERD)**
3. **Respiratory system (wheezing)**

What age group most often develops "milk allergy?"

Infants
(<2 years old)

What is the natural course of milk allergy?

It usually resolves spontaneously

Is it possible to develop milk allergy if the infant is exclusively breast fed?

Yes –
Proteins may be passed through the mother's milk

(*Maternal avoidance of milk & beef products is helpful*)

How common is milk allergy in infants?

Common
(about 1 in 20)

Why might a child with milk protein allergy develop anemia?

Occult blood loss

(due to low-level allergic colitis)

How is a milk allergy diagnosis usually made?

Removal of milk products produces clinical improvement

What is the best initial formula choice for a milk allergy infant? Why?

• **Hydrolyzed formulas**
• **Milk allergy kids are often also allergic to soy**

When milk products are removed from a child's diet, how fast should improvement occur, if the problem was milk allergy?

Blood in stool should be gone in less than 3 days

(complete resolution may take 2 weeks, especially for breast fed infants)

What are the histologic findings of milk allergy (in the gut)?
(3)

1. Villous atrophy
2. Increased lymphocytes
3. Eosinophilia (in the gut wall)

How is the outcome of acute pancreatitis different from that of chronic pancreatitis?

Pancreatic form & function usually go back to normal with <u>acute</u>

When does fat and protein malabsorption become a problem, as a consequence of exocrine pancreatic function?

When *90%* of exocrine function is lost

How do patients with acute pancreatitis *usually* present?
(4)

1. **Abdominal pain**
2. **Nausea & vomiting**
3. **Pain radiates to back**
4. **± Low-grade temp**

What are two mechanical causes of pancreatitis in children?

Trauma

&

Outflow obstruction
(including congenital structural problems & gallstones)

What three causes of pancreatitis in kids are based on inflammatory reactions?

1. Drugs
2. Reflux of bile
3. Infection/systemic diseases

In general, will children with pancreatitis do better, or worse, than adults?

Better
(low mortality)

What lung problems sometimes accompany pancreatitis?
(2)

Pleural effusion & ARDS

What calcium disorder are pancreatitis patients likely to develop?

Hypocalcemia
(about 15 %)

How good is a serum amylase at identifying pancreatitis?

Not good
(most hollow structures, plus some tumors, etc., elevate amylase)

What lab test is more helpful than amylase in specifically identifying pancreatitis & pancreatic injury?

Lipase

Which radiological study is best for evaluating possible pancreatitis?

Contrast CT

What are the main ways we treat pancreatitis patients?
(4)

1. **NPO (bowel rest) with early resumption of enteral feeding**
2. **NG tube (initial bowel rest & vomiting)**
3. **IV fluids!!!**
4. **Appropriate pain management**

A child who complains of chronic abdominal pain, who also has asthma and recurrent bouts of sinusitis, should be worked up for what problem?

Cystic fibrosis

Child – asthma – sinusitis – abdominal pain (chronic) = what diagnosis?

CF

What is the usual cause of significant abdominal pain in CF patients, when the abdominal pain is related to the CF?

Pancreatitis

What abdominal X-ray findings suggest pancreatitis?
(3 main findings)

1. **Sentinel loop (widened bowel loop near pancreas)**
2. **Ileus**
3. **Calcifications in the pancreas (chronic pancreatitis only)**

What syndrome of three related problems runs in families with "hereditary pancreatitis?"

1. Diabetes mellitus
2. Recurrent pancreatitis
3. Pancreatic cancer

Hemorrhagic pancreatitis presents a little differently on the lab tests, compared to regular pancreatitis. How is it different?

Hgb *either low* (due to loss in the abdomen)

Or

high (due to hemoconcentration with third spacing)

How does a perirectal abscess usually get it start?

Infection in anal gland

What chronic complication may result from a perirectal abscess?

Fistula (!)

Why are perirectal abscesses a "big deal"?

If not treated promptly, they can spread in *any* direction

Perianal abscesses may also look like what noninfectious problem?

Thrombosed external hemorrhoid

Who takes care of a perirectal abscess?

Usually best done by a surgeon (due to potential spread into areas you may not appreciate)

How common is fistula formation with a perirectal abscess?

Common
(about 25 %)

Will a perirectal abscess recur?

No –
Unless it was due to IBD or another chronic condition

What is a perirectal abscess called, if it spreads horizontally into the perineal area?

Ischiorectal abscess –
Often produces sepsis!

Should you prescribe antibiotics for perirectal abscesses?

Not usually –
I&D should be sufficient

What is the most common organism to cause perirectal abscesses?

Staphylococcus aureus

In what situations *would* you give antibiotics for a perirectal abscess? (4 situations)

1. Systemically ill
2. Immunocompromised
3. Extensive cellulitis
4. Valvular heart disease

Which IBD is associated with perirectal abscess?

Crohn's disease

What does "spontaneous bacterial peritonitis" mean?

There was no intra-abdominal infection source
(for example, ruptured gut, abscess)

Which patients are most at risk for SBP?

Those with ascites (especially if they have cirrhosis)

Why are patients with ascites more at risk for SBP?

1. Poor phagocyte activity

2. Less filtering of blood in liver if cirrhotic

3. Complement is decreased in the ascitic fluid (making phagocytes less effective)

Are most SBP pathogens aerobic or anaerobic?

<u>Aerobic</u>

Are most SBP pathogens Gram negative or Gram positive?

<u>Negative</u>

What other body fluid is often positive for the same organism as the ascitic fluid?

Urine
(in at least 1/3 of cases)

What is the prognosis for SBP?

Alright –
Few die if appropriate antibiotics (generally third-generation cephalosporins or sometimes fluoroquinolones) are started before shock or renal failure develop

If your patient survives a bout of SBP, is it likely to recur?

Yes –
At least 50 % have another episode

What is the prognosis over a 1–2-year period, for a patient who has had SBP?

Low (around 20 %) *due to their overall poor health & limited liver function*

Can SBP be asymptomatic?

Yes
(about 10 %)

Which type of bacterial peritonitis is more likely to have ascitic fluid with high LDH & protein and low glucose?

Secondary bacterial peritonitis

(holes in the gut often elevate LDH)

Spontaneous bacterial peritonitis fluid should grow out only one organism. In secondary bacterial peritonitis, what do you expect the culture to show?

Polymicrobial gut organisms

What is the best early indicator of SBP, in terms of ascites labs?

High PMN count
($>250/\text{mm}^3$)

What are three potentially life-threatening complications of bacterial peritonitis?

1. Sepsis

2. Respiratory compromise (due to rapidly increasing fluid)

3. Hypovolemia (due to third spacing)

What proportion of infants with necrotizing enterocolitis is full term?

About 10 %

(more than you would think! Often they have cardiac or other conditions)

What part(s) of the gut are typically affected by NEC?

Terminal ileum
Ileocecal region
Ascending colon

What is usually seen, histologically, in NEC lesions?

(2)

Inflammation

&

Coagulation necrosis

What is the relationship between NEC and birth weight?

1. **Lower birth weights are more likely to get it**
2. **The lower the birth weight, the longer the infant is at risk**

What is the relationship between types of feedings and onset of NEC?

95 % of NEC infants develop NEC after enteral feeds are started

What is the NEC triad of signs?
(of course, not all patients display the triad)

1. **Bilious emesis**
2. **Bloody stools**
3. **Abdominal distention**

What X-ray finding is most associated with NEC?

Pneumatosis intestinalis

(and gas in the hepatic venous system)

If the infant recovers from NEC, what gut problems often remain?

Strictures & short gut syndrome
(if the infant had surgery)

What is a pancreatic pseudocyst?

A fibrous capsule without a true epithelium (attached to the pancreas)

What usually leads to pancreatic pseudocyst formation in kids?

Trauma leads to inflammation, then pseudocyst formation

Should pancreatic pseudocyst patients have high pancreatic enzyme levels?

Sometimes –
If the cyst is open to the pancreatic duct system, the levels will be elevated

If a pancreatic pseudocyst patient does not have elevated enzyme levels, what does that mean?

The pseudocyst is not open to the rest of the pancreas

What happens to pseudocysts if left alone?

Spontaneous resolution (assuming that they don't rupture)

What symptoms do pancreatic pseudocyst patients often have?
(3)

1. **Pain**
2. **Nausea/vomiting**
3. **Weight loss**

What radiological modality is most preferred for the identification of pancreatic pseudocysts?

CT

(ultrasound is also used, and is handy for screening, but provides less info)

Is it safe to perform an ERCP on patients with pancreatic pseudocyst, to evaluate the pseudocysts?

(ERCP = endoscopic retrograde cholangiopancreatography)

Usually, if:

Broad-spectrum antibiotics are used

&

A definitive procedure to correct the cysts is planned within 24 h

Which pancreatic pseudocysts are most concerning?

1. **Symptomatic**
2. **>6 cm**
3. **Increasing size** (especially if >6 cm)

If a pseudocyst requires drainage, how can that be accomplished?

1. Open surgical drainage

2. Percutaneous drainage

3. Endoscopic stent placement

4. Endoscopic surgery

What vascular system complications are sometimes seen with pancreatic pseudocyst?

IVC or splenic vein obstruction
(due to pressure on & inflammation of the vein from the cyst)

&

Hemorrhage
(usually due to an associated pseudoaneurysm)

How is a pancreatic pseudocyst treated if it becomes infected?

Immediate (external) drainage

What is the usual cause of pseudocyst formation in children?

Traumatic pancreatitis

How common is pseudocyst rupture?

Uncommon
(<10 %)

How worrisome is a pseudocyst rupture?

Quite worrisome –
If hemorrhage or pus is involved, mortality is significant

In addition to obstructing the IVC, what other "mechanical" problems do pseudocysts cause?

Obstruction of <u>any</u> of the abdominal organs & systems

(biliary, portal venous, urinary, colonic, etc.)

Pressure of the (venous) blood in the portal system is regulated by what two factors?

Volume of blood

&

Resistance

What unusual feature in the portal venous system allows varices to form?

There are no valves

(the pressure gradient therefore determines flow)

Why does portal hypertension sometimes lead to malabsorption of nutrients?

Venous congestion of mucosa

(can be so severe that gut absorption is compromised)

What is the most common presenting symptom of portal hypertension?

Esophageal variceal hemorrhage

What are the three general ways that portal hypertension usually develops?

1. **Suprahepatic (above the liver)**
2. **Infrahepatic**
3. **Subhepatic**

What are some typical causes of suprahepatic portal hypertension?

**Budd–Chiari
(clot just above the liver)**

&

Congestive heart failure

Do suprahepatic problems cause portal hypertension often?

No –
Only about 10 % of cases are suprahepatic etiologies

Which general type of portal hypertension is most common?

<u>Intrahepatic</u>

(about 60 %)

What are some typical causes of intrahepatic portal hypertension?
(6)

1. **Cirrhosis (all causes & types)**
2. **Schistosomiasis**
3. **Vitamin A toxicity**
4. **Peliosis hepatitis (androgen related)**
5. **Congenital fibrosis**
6. **Wilson disease**

Subhepatic portal hypertension can occur when what two vessels occlude?

Splenic vein

Or

Portal vein

What special complication are patients at risk for if they have a stoma, and also develop portal hypertension?

Stomal variceal bleeding

(threatens the airway!!!)

Will the size of the spleen correlate well to the portal pressure?

No

(Splenomegaly is suggestive of portal hypertension, but the size does not relate to the pressure well)

Prominent abdominal vessels in the setting of portal hypertension have what special name?

Caput medusa

(head of medusa – medusa had hair made of snakes in the Greek myth)

In portal hypertension, should the liver be large, small, or normal sized?

Could be any of the them – depends on the problem

In a stable patient, what is the test of choice to evaluate the cause (and effects) of portal hypertension?

Ultrasound with doppler

What is "hepatofugal flow," and what does it indicate?

- **Flow away from the liver**
- **Likely portal hypertension or other obstruction**

How can an EGD be useful in a portal hypertension patient?

To evaluate varices & treat bleeding

What techniques are available to the endoscopist to treat bleeding esophageal varices?
(2)

Ligation

&

Sclerotherapy

What is a hepatic venous wedge pressure used for, and is it often used in pediatric liver patients?

- In adults, it correlates well with bleeding risk
- Not frequently used in kids – not clear whether it's useful

How useful is a barium swallow in detecting varices?

Okay, but not great –
80–90 % sensitivity & specificity

What temporary mechanical tool is available to manage variceal bleeding?

The Sengstaken–Blakemore tube

(tube that goes into the esophagus and inflates to apply direct pressure)

What medications are most commonly used in the management of variceal bleeding?
(3)

1. **Vasopressin (constricts splanchnic vessels)**
2. **Somatostatin**
3. **Nitroglycerin (lowers venous tone)**

In addition to the use of blood products, in general, what might you specifically need to give to bleeding portal hypertension patients?

Fresh frozen plasma

&

Vitamin K
(their livers may not be working well, yielding coagulopathy)

How can β-blockers be useful in portal hypertension?

- **They decrease cardiac output, reducing delivery of blood to the system**
- **β₂ blockade increases resistance in the vessels, decreasing blood in the portal system**

What special danger limits the use of β-blockers in portal hypertension patients?

They blunt the cardiovascular response needed if there is a big bleed

How successful is liver transplantation as a treatment for most forms of portal hypertension?

Better than any other approach

Should sclerotherapy be used to prevent bleeding from varices?

**No –
Data supports its use to prevent <u>recurrent</u> bleeding but not first-time bleeding**

What are the main indications for liver transplantation in a portal hypertension patient?
(3)

1. Growth failure
2. Life-threatening bleeds
3. Unacceptable quality of life

What is the utility of NG lavage in upper GI bleeding?

1. **Confirms bleed is upper GI (although if the patient has hematemesis, you already know that)**

2. **Some say that it is therapeutic (not clear how)**

Is surgical shunting a good option for pediatric portal hypertension patients?

Usually not –
Rex shunts can be used for extrahepatic causes (usually following liver transplant), & some success with TiPS is now reported

Most infants with pyloric stenosis are completely normal otherwise – what abnormalities are sometimes associated with pyloric stenosis, though?
(2)

Esophageal atresia

&

Malrotation (with short gut)

What is pyloric stenosis?

Pyloric hypertrophy producing gastric outflow obstruction

When does pyloric stenosis most often present?

Around 4 weeks
(can be shortly after birth to a few months later, but around 4 weeks is most common)

What should you be able to palpate on an infant with pyloric stenosis?

An "olive" in the right epigastrium

(you are feeling the hypertrophied pylorus itself)

If an infant with pyloric stenosis has just eaten, what might you observe on physical exam?

Visible peristalsis

(from the left upper quadrant toward the pylorus)

What does "string sign" refer to?

The appearance of the narrow pyloric canal on barium swallow

In addition to "string sign," what other barium swallow finding indicates pyloric stenosis?

"Train tracks"

(narrow, double stripes of barium)

Why might ultrasound be a better diagnostic modality for pyloric stenosis than barium upper GI?	No risk of aspiration
If ultrasound is used to diagnose pyloric stenosis, what findings make the diagnosis?	Muscle thickness >4 mm Or Pyloric length >14 mm
What pH and electrolyte abnormalities would you expect in a vomiting pyloric stenosis baby?	**pH – alkalotic (vomiting out the stomach acid)** **Chloride – low** **Potassium – low (renal mechanism)** **Sodium – low or sometimes high**
Why is the chloride often so low in pyloric stenosis babies?	**They are losing it directly in the stomach acid (HCl) they vomit**
How is pyloric stenosis managed?	**Medical management of pH and electrolyte abnormalities, *then* surgical correction**
How should you replace the chloride lost in pyloric stenosis patients?	**With normal saline** **(corrects volume, sodium, *and* chloride)**
What is the name of the surgical procedure to correct pyloric stenosis?	Ramstedt (pyloromyotomy) procedure
If a pyloric stenosis infant has definitive surgery and then continues to vomit, what does that indicate?	Usually just post-op swelling – will spontaneously resolve in a few days
How is the Ramstedt procedure to correct pyloric stenosis performed?	An incision is made in the antro-pyloric muscle
Is pyloric stenosis thought to have a genetic or an environmental cause?	Both contribute – Full etiology is not known
What is a complete rectal prolapse?	**All rectal layers emerge from the anus**
What worrisome gut complication only occurs when the rectal prolapse is complete?	**Bowel strangulation –** ***Gut & peritoneum may also come through***

What is a "concealed" rectal prolapse?	Intussusception of the upper rectum into the lower portion – Nothing shows externally
What does "incomplete" rectal prolapse mean?	**Only** the mucosal layers prolapse
How might malnutrition contribute to rectal prolapse?	Loss of the ischiorectal fat pad in very thin individuals makes prolapse more likely
What types of bowel habits are thought to contribute to prolapse?	**Both constipation/straining & diarrhea**
Which three patient groups are most likely to suffer from rectal prolapse?	1. Females 2. Cystic fibrosis patients (especially <2 years old) 3. Patients living in less developed countries
What are the typical complications of rectal prolapse?	1. **Proctitis** 2. **Rectal ulcers (not very common)** 3. **Painless rectal bleeding**
How is rectal prolapse usually treated?	**Spontaneously reduces** **(or is easily reduced manually)**
If you see a prolapse on physical exam, how can you tell whether it's complete or incomplete?	• Incomplete should have a radial pattern (like spokes on a bicycle wheel) • Complete has concentric circles (more like a target)
What do you typically see on physical exam of a rectal prolapse patient?	**Nothing –** **It's usually gone by the time you see the patient, because it spontaneously reduces when they're not straining**
What medication is of great help in decreasing rectal prolapse for CF patients?	**Pancreatic enzyme supplementation**
When surgery is used to correct recurrent rectal prolapse, how likely are complications?	Very likely

What is the main complication of surgical correction for recurrent rectal prolapse?	Constipation
What are the two main contributing factors you should rule out in a child presenting for rectal prolapse?	**Cystic fibrosis** **&** **Constipation**
Which pediatric patients develop short bowel syndrome?	**Those who have had small bowel resections are at risk** **(They don't all develop it, though)**
Why do infants have more difficulty, in the short term, with small bowel resection than older children or adults do?	**Infants have less "gut reserve" (because their bowel length is short)**
There are three underlying reasons for short bowel syndrome. What are they?	1. **Abnormal (rapid) transit time** 2. **Nutrient malabsorption (depends on which part of the bowel is missing)** 3. **Decreased mucosal surface**
In addition to the syndrome, itself, what other complications are all short bowel patients at risk for?	1. Gastric acid hypersecretion (transient – follows the surgery) 2. *Bacterial overgrowth* 3. Renal stones 4. Gallstones
In general terms, why does having a short bowel make you more likely to have kidney stones?	Changes in absorption pattern increase stone formation (Fat malabsorption & high oxalate absorption)
Why would a short bowel patient be more likely to make gall stones?	Changes in the enterohepatic recirculation pathway increase stone formation
Why are children with short bowel syndrome likely to have perianal rashes?	**Stool is often acidic**

Are antidiarrheal medications helpful in short bowel syndrome?	Yes – They (usually) decrease motility (increased risk of bacterial overgrowth, though)
There are two other types of medications that are helpful in controlling the diarrhea of short bowel syndrome. What are they?	Octreotide (decreases secretions & motility) & Ion-exchange resins (bind bile acids, so they don't contribute to diarrhea)
When might a <u>pro</u>kinetic medication be helpful in short bowel syndrome?	Patients with: Bile reflux Or Pseudoobstruction (*cisapride is commonly used – watch out for QTc prolongation!*)
How are H_2 blockers helpful in short bowel syndrome? (3 mechanisms)	1. Decrease acid (if needed) 2. Decrease secretory volume overall 3. Decrease sodium & potassium losses
How are "intestinal interpositions" used to surgically increase absorption?	The added bowel helps to slow transit (sometimes it is placed in reverse orientation for *backward* peristalsis)
How does the bowel "adapt" after shortening?	• May dilate & lengthen • Villi may hypertrophy (increases surface area)
Which portion of the gut is most able to adapt after shortening?	The ileum
How much bowel must remain for a good prognosis, in an infant with short bowel?	$\geq 10\%$ of predicted small bowel length for age
If the ileocecal valve must be removed, it decreases the chances that a short bowel patient will be able to reach what important goal?	Independence from parenteral nutrition

Which gut segment is mainly responsible for absorption of protein?

Jejunum

What segment(s) of gut is/are mainly responsible for absorption of fat?

Stomach

&

Ileum

What general factors are most predictive of how well a patient will do after a significant bowel resection?

(4)

1. **Size of resection (bigger is worse)**
2. **Loss of ileocecal valve is worse**
3. **Loss of ileum or jejunum worse**
4. **Length of time until successful enteral feeds (shorter is better)**

Where are most minerals & metals absorbed?

Duodenum
(calcium, magnesium, iron, & zinc)

What important items does the ileum absorb?

(3)

Fat
Bile salts
Vitamin B12 (!)

In addition to protein, what is the jejunum responsible for absorbing?

(3)

1. Water-soluble vitamins
2. Fat-soluble vitamins A & D
3. Mono & disaccharides (simple sugars)

In addition to absorption of fluid, what other important absorptive functions are done by the colon?

Electrolytes

&

Short-chain fatty acids

What problems does TPN sometimes cause for the liver?

(3)

1. *Cholestasis*
2. **Portal hypertension**
3. **Cirrhosis**

TPN is important in the early stages of recovery from bowel resection. How is TPN sometimes related to bad outcomes for these patients?

TPN liver disease can develop

(severe disease is a *bad* prognostic & combined liver–small bowel transplant can sometimes be necessary)

What is the common name for the liver disease syndrome that sometimes develops in patients requiring parenteral nutrition?

Parenteral nutrition liver disease – PNLD

The lactose breath test checks for lactase deficiency. What does the <u>lactulose</u> breath test look for?

Bacterial overgrowth

What is superior mesenteric artery syndrome?

Duodenal obstruction due to pressure from the SMA

How is SMA syndrome definitively treated?

It usually resolves spontaneously

Why does back surgery or spinal abnormality contribute to the incidence of SMA syndrome?

The duodenum is caught between the SMA anteriorly and the vertebra posteriorly

What are the main symptoms of SMA syndrome?
(4)

1. Vomiting (bilious or not)
2. Abdominal pain
3. Early satiety
4. Bloating

What might abdominal radiography show in SMA syndrome?

Dilated bowel proximal to the SMA, then sharp cutoff

What fairly simple intervention can you try to improve feeding for SMA syndrome patients?
(4)

1. Feed while prone or left lateral position
2. Decrease viscosity
3. J-tube (jejunal tube)
4. Body cast patients can be repositioned often

When surgery is necessary for SMA syndrome, what is the usual outcome?

Good
(There are several procedures)

Is "toddler's diarrhea" an infectious disease?

No

What are the basic criteria for diagnosing toddler's diarrhea?
(3)

• **Child aged 1–5 years** (some sources say 6 months, but that's not a toddler!)

• **Diarrhea lasting 3–4 weeks**

• **Child is otherwise well**

What are the three likely causes of toddler's diarrhea?

1. **Too much fruit juice (excess fructose & sorbitol)**
2. **High fluid, low fat & fiber**
3. **Motility disorder**

Toddler's diarrhea often follows what type of problem?	**Acute gastroenteritis (complicated by high carb diets followed due to the gastritis)**
What is the most common cause of long-term diarrhea, without FTT, in young children?	**Toddler's diarrhea**
Toddler's diarrhea often occurs in families with members suffering from what GI problem?	Functional bowel disorders (interesting …)
In toddler's diarrhea, what is the usual description of the stool?	**Foul smelling** **&** **Contains undigested food particles** (both are due to very rapid transit)
How is toddler's diarrhea treated, and how fast will it respond?	• **Alter diet (less fluid, less juice, more fat & fiber)** • **Days to weeks**
Are medications suggested for treatment of toddler's diarrhea?	**Only in refractory cases** (loperamide used when needed)
When should a toddler's diarrhea patient be referred for specialist consultation? **(3 situations)**	1. **No response to diet modification** *after 2 weeks* 2. **Growth is affected** 3. **Other complaints develop**
Why is the fructose in juice especially difficult for the gut to absorb?	There is a glucose–fructose co-transporter that allows easier absorption of fructose if an equal amount of glucose is present (Excess fructose, compared to the amount of glucose, overwhelms this system)
What is the most common congenital problem with the esophagus?	Atresia/TEF
What proportion of children with TEF (tracheoesophageal fistula) has associated anomalies?	**50 %** (most often cardiac)

What are the three general types of TEF?	1. **Proximal TEF (may also have a distal TEF)**
	2. **Distal TEF**
	3. **H-type (no esophageal atresia)**
What type of TEF is most common?	**Distal TEF (about 90 %)**
Why is the "H-type" of TEF named "H-type?"	**It is the only type of TEF without esophageal atresia. The parallel esophagus & trachea, with a connecting fistula, make an "H" shape**
Does esophageal atresia without TEF also occur?	Yes (much less common, though – about 5 % of all infants with esophageal errors of development)
How do TEFs occur?	The foregut is divided into trachea & esophagus by a septum – *Incomplete division → a TEF*
At what point in development does a TEF form?	Early – 4–8 weeks gestation
What percentage of children with TEF has the VATER or VACTERL syndrome?	10 %
What proportion of esophageal atresia patients *without fistula* will develop polyhydramnios?	80 % (not 100 %)
What pulmonary complications commonly occur with TEF? **(3)**	1. **Respiratory distress** 2. **Pneumonia (usually lower lobes)** 3. **Chronic cough (foreign body impaction)**
What special danger is present for TEF infants on a ventilator?	Gastric perforation
What complication is even more likely than usual to occur with endotracheal intubation of an infant with a TEF?	Distension of abdominal viscera (by air)

If you need to intubate a TEF patient, what special considerations should you think about?

(2)

- Tip should be below fistula (but above carina)
- Bevelled edge of the tube should be facing the chest wall (less gas will enter stomach)

If 80 % of esophageal atresia infants have polyhydramnios, what proportion of TEF infants will have polyhydramnios?

About 30 %

(and 1/3 are born prematurely)

Why are TEF patients with distal fistulas still at risk for pneumonia or other respiratory problems?

Esophageal dysmotility and reflux

(can still cause damage to the pulmonary system)

The prognostic categories for TEF patients consider which preoperative items?

(2)

Ventilator dependence

&

Anomalies – none, major, or minor

A chronic cough, with recurrent aspiration-type pneumonia, and intermittent wheezing may indicate what type of TEF?

H-type

What is the "classic" TEF presentation?

(3)

- **Emesis of feeds**
- **Cyanosis/choking with feeds**
- **Excessive salivation/drooling from birth**

What simple bedside test is helpful in diagnosing TEF or esophageal atresia?

**NG tube –
Can't advance it beyond 10 cm or so**

What radiological evaluations are helpful in evaluating a possible TEF?

- **Contrast esophagogram**
- **Bronchoscopy/esophagoscopy**

In addition to imaging of the trachea & esophagus, what other radiological studies might you want to consider in a TEF patient?

(3)

Rule out associated abnormalities:

- **Echocardiogram**
- **Renal ultrasound**
- **X-rays of limbs & vertebra**

How will esophageal atresia (with or without fistula) look on X-ray? (3 findings)	1. Coiled-up feeding tube 2. Air-distended stomach 3. No air in the stomach
When admitting a TEF infant, what initial measures do you need to take? (4 items)	1. **NG suction** 2. **Aspiration precautions (elevate head of bed)** 3. **Peds surgery consult (emergency ligation of the fistula is sometimes required)** 4. **Prophylactic antibiotics, if surgery will be soon**
What does a primary TEF repair entail?	**Esophageal anastomosis (if the gap is <3 cm)** **&** **Division of fistula (of course)**
When is the primary repair for a TEF usually done?	First 2 days of life
How is a delayed TEF repair different from a primary repair?	Initially – Fistula is ligated & gastrostomy performed Within 30 days – Delayed primary anastomosis
What makes a TEF repair "staged" rather than "delayed?"	Definitive surgery more than 30 days after the initial procedure is "staged"
When is primary repair for TEF or esophageal atresia usually not done? (3 situations)	• Significant respiratory distress • Isolated esophageal atresia • Long-gap atresia (>3 cm)
What is "cervical esophagostomy" used for?	AKA a "spit fistula" • Allows saliva to escape for patients with frequent aspiration • Temporizing measure for patients who require esophageal replacement (anastomosis not possible)

Although the outcome for infants with TEF is usually good, what complications are possible?

(3 specific ones)

1. Stricture or leak at the surgical anastomosis
2. Refistulization
3. GERD

When might post-op paralysis & mechanical ventilation be recommended for post-op TEF patients?

(For up to 7 days!)

If the repair is under significant tension (*long-gap repair*)

What complications is a period of mechanical ventilation intended to prevent in long-gap repair?

Reflux

&

Stricture formation

Why should you be very conservative about removing the ET tube after a TEF repair?

Reintubation has a significant chance of rupturing the trachea (at the repair site)

When is it alright to feed a post-op TEF patient orally and remove the chest tube/drain?

When the anastomosis is shown to be healed & patent on contrast swallow study

Why is a partial gastric fundoplication needed in most TEF patients?

Usually have bad reflux

How common are post-op anastomotic leaks, following TEF repair?

Common (15 %) –

most close spontaneously in 1–2 weeks!

How good is prenatal ultrasound at identifying a TEF?

Not good –
Identifies only about 10 % with an 18-week ultrasound

Is TEF an inherited disorder?

There is probably a small genetic component but no clear inheritance pattern

Are the lesions of ulcerative colitis continuous or "skip lesions?"

Continuous!

(Skip lesions = Crohn's)

What part of the gut does ulcerative colitis (UC) affect?

**It begins at the rectum & works its way backward –
Can affect all of the colon, but usually stays on the left**

What are the genetics of UC?

Clear familial groupings, & associated with various HLA types

What is the buzzword for ulcerative colitis on histological evaluation?

Crypt abscesses

Ulcerative colitis patients are at increased risk of adenocarcinoma after how many years?

10 years after disease onset

What other disorders are UC patients at increased risk to develop?

- **Primary sclerosing cholangitis**
- **Kidney stones**
- **Uveitis, arthritis, & spondylitis**

What are the most common presenting signs/symptoms of UC?

- **Abdominal pain & rectal bleeding – 90 %**
- **Diarrhea – 50 %**

Will ulcerative colitis patients present with fever?

Yes, often –
Usually low grade

If a patient presents with bloody diarrhea, but his or her symptoms have been present for less than 3 weeks, should UC be at the top of the differential?

No –
Think infectious first

When should colonoscopy be avoided in UC patients?

Severe episodes (fulminant)

Likely to perforate

What percentage of UC patients are positive for pANCA?

About 70 %

(25 % of Crohn's are also positive)

Why might a UC patient develop anemia?
(2 reasons)

Chronic GI bleeding
&
Poor iron absorption

What is the ASCA test, and with which GI disorder is it associated?

- Anti-saccharomyces cerevisiae antibody (ASCA)
- Crohn's disease (& to a lesser extent with ulcerative colitis)

What are the three options for treating mild UC?	1. **Topical 5-ASA** 2. **Sulfasalazine** 3. **Corticosteroids**
How is moderately severe UC treated? (4 components)	1. **Sulfasalazine** 2. **IV steroids (short term)** 3. **Low-residue diet** 4. **± Oral antibiotics**
How is severe UC treated? (3 main components)	1. **IV steroids** 2. **No diet (bowel rest)** 3. **Triple IV antibiotics**
When are immunosuppressive medications, other than steroids, indicated for UC?	**Usually if regular therapy has failed after a 2-week period**
How high should you keep the ANC (absolute neutrophil count) in an immunosuppressed UC patient?	Above 500
Which immunosuppressive medication is usually used to induce remission in refractory UC patients?	**Cyclosporine** Mnemonic: UC comes in "cycles." Cyclosporine *cycles* you into remission
Which immunosuppressive agents can be used to *maintain* remission?	**6-mercaptopurine** & **Azathioprine**
Why is folate usually given to IBD patients?	**Sulfasalazine impairs its absorption** **(so we give extra to make up for the poor absorption)**
What special blood test should you check before starting sulfasalazine therapy?	**G6PD deficiency** **(The sulfa moiety will induce RBC lysis)**
When surgery is needed for pediatric UC patients, what procedure is usually performed?	Ileoanal anastomosis

When is surgery for UC performed urgently or emergently?
(4 situations)

1. **If toxic megacolon has developed**
2. **Perforation**
3. **Significant bleeding**
4. **Fulminant colitis failing medical therapy**

If toxic megacolon is diagnosed, what are the initial management steps?
(4)

1. **NPO**
2. **No GI procedures**
3. **No antimotility meds (including anticholinergics, narcotics)**
4. **Broad-spectrum antibiotics**

What is the guiding principle in managing toxic megacolon?

AVOID PERFORATION

If perforation has <u>not</u> occurred, why might you still consider surgery for toxic megacolon?

Failure of medical therapy after 24–72 h

(due to high risk of perforation & sepsis as time goes by)

Why can toxic megacolon cause complications even if the colon does *not* perforate?

The colonic barrier to toxins & bacteria breaks down, allowing them to escape into the circulation

How is toxic megacolon diagnosed?

Part or all of colon dilated to ≥6 cm in adolescents and adults

Which general type of colitis is most likely to lead to toxic megacolon?

Pancolitis

Does mechanical manipulation of the colon increase the risk of developing toxic megacolon?

Yes –
Recent barium enema or scoping does

Are UC patients at more risk for toxic megacolon when they have many repeated episodes, or during their first episode of UC?

First episode

Use of which two medication classes are linked to increased incidence of toxic megacolon?

Opiates
    &
Anticholinergics

What is the main problem in Reye's syndrome (in terms of the pathophysiology)?	**Enzymes of liver mitochondria are somehow significantly reduced**
What medication significantly worsens the pathophysiology of Reye's syndrome?	**Aspirin** **(It's not clear what happens – ASA is only harmful if ingested *after* the mitochondrial injury)**
What histologic change is seen in the liver with Reye's syndrome?	Fatty degeneration
Which viruses are most associated with the development of Reye's syndrome?	**Varicella** **&** **Influenza A & B**
What is the typical Reye's syndrome patient profile? (3 characteristics)	• White • 6 years old (4–12 years) • <u>Not</u> a city kid
What is the average mortality for Reye's syndrome?	About 20 % (was about 40 %, but recognition seems to have improved!)
Which type of hepatitis sometimes precedes Reye's syndrome?	Hepatitis A
In addition to the liver, what other organ is significantly affected in Reye's syndrome?	The brain
Will a Reye's syndrome patient have focal neurological findings?	No
How does Reye's syndrome present in its early phases?	• **Sudden onset vomiting** • **Mild cognitive & behavioral changes**
What problems occur in the brains of Reye's syndrome patients?	• **Abnormal mitochondria** • **Edema** • **Elevated ICP**

When treating a Reye's syndrome patient, what two complications of the liver dysfunction will you need to treat?

Hypoglycemia
(give glucose – glycogen stores are gone)

&

Coagulopathy
(give FFP & vitamin K, as needed)

What is the best predictor of final outcome for Reye's syndrome patients?

Cerebral function at presentation

What is the usual cause of death for those Reye's patients that do not survive?

Cerebral edema

What is intestinal volvulus?

**Rotation of the gut
(or mesentery)**

When gut rotates, it usually causes obstruction. In volvulus, is this obstruction chronic or acute?

**Can be either –
Chronic volvulus usually causes an intermittent problem**

Which pediatric patients are most likely to develop volvulus?

Infants/neonates with malrotation

Why might volvulus patients develop "chylous ascites" or protein-losing enteropathy?

Lymphatic congestion

What age group most often develops volvulus, amongst pediatric patients?

Neonates

What might you see on the abdominal X-ray of a volvulus patient?
(3 possibilities)

- Dilated stomach/duodenum
- Cecum in the upper quadrant
- Corkscrew or Z-shaped duodenum

What metabolic derangement often occurs in ischemic gut?

Metabolic acidosis

(Ischemic tissue gets acidotic!)

What is the name of the surgical procedure used to correct midgut volvulus and prevent it from happening again?

The "Ladd" procedure

What is one tipoff that emesis may be the result of volvulus or other obstruction?

It is bilious

What two benign tumors of the salivary gland often occur during infancy?

Hemangioma

&

Lymphangioma
(aka cystic hygroma)

How are salivary hemangiomas treated?

Usually they involute spontaneously

(If they don't, steroids are injected into them)

How are salivary lymphangiomas treated?

Surgical resection
(if it will not damage the facial nerve, of course – steroids, radiation, or sclerotherapy may be tried if surgery is not an option)

What is the most common salivary gland tumor to develop from epithelial cells, and which patients develop it?

- Benign mixed tumor

- Adolescent girls

What is the significance of isolated colonic polyps in children?

Usually no significance

What embryological problem causes cleft lip?

(*popular test item!*)

**Failure of fusion:
Maxillary & medial nasal processes**

What embryological problem causes cleft palate?

(*popular test item!*)

**Failure of fusion:
Palatal "shelves"**

Which two ethnic groups have the highest rate of cleft lip & palate?

Native Americans & Asians

Which happens more often, cleft lip or cleft palate?

Cleft lip

(by a lot!)

Which ethnic group has the *lowest* rate of cleft lip or palate?

African Americans

What is the most minimal type of cleft palate?	Bifid (divided) uvula
Are the teeth involved in cleft lip?	Sometimes – The alveolar ridge can be involved
How can you have a "bilateral" cleft lip?	There are two medial nasal processes – If *both fail to fuse*, it is bilateral

How is cleft lip treated?
                    (4)

1. Surgical repair
2. Speech therapy
3. Dentistry/orthodontics
4. Pressure equalization tubes to treat effusions & protect hearing, if needed

What is the first problem infants with cleft lip develop?	Difficulty feeding

How is the surgical repair of cleft lip & palate done, in general terms?

In stages:

- Lip is repaired first (by 3 months old)

- Palatal repair by 12 months

What helps infants with cleft lip/palate to feed more easily?
                    (3)

- Soft, large, artificial nipples

- Squeezable bottles

- Upright feeding (gravity helps the milk go down)

Some reflux is very common in infants. At what age is reflux most common?	4 months

**What are the main signs
of problematic infant reflux?**
                    (3)

- **Arching the body**
- **Choking/gagging**
- **Feeding aversion**

    (+ Irritability – you'd be irritable, too, if it hurts whenever you eat!)

By what age does infant reflux usually resolve?	2 years

What are "atypical" signs of GERD? (4)	• Chest pain • Pulmonary – Asthma/cough/ bronchitis • Laryngeal – Hoarseness/laryngitis • Tooth decay
Do patients with atypical GERD have typical symptoms, also?	Usually not
Although most patients with hiatal hernia are asymptomatic, how does hiatal hernia contribute to GERD? (Two mechanisms)	May make the LES less functional (messes up the mechanics) & Often traps some gastric contents up high, making reflux more likely
What are the three general ways that reflux happens?	1. Less resistance to esophageal reflux than usual (hernia or sphincter problem) 2. Decreased clearance (bad peristalsis) 3. Gastric or lower gut problems
Is extensive testing needed to diagnose GERD (especially in older children or adults)?	No – Usually a clinical diagnosis
What are "typical" GERD complaints?	• **Heartburn (worse lying down, worse after meals)** • **Painful swallowing** • **Regurgitation/acid taste**
If you are not certain of a GERD diagnosis, what is the typical way to verify it?	**Empiric trial of proton pump inhibitors**
What radiological study is helpful in diagnosing GERD and its complications?	Barium esophagogram (can see the reflux of barium + hernias, obstruction, stricture, etc.)
If a patient has atypical GERD symptoms, what will help you to guess that GERD might be the cause?	The atypical symptoms often follow typical GERD triggers

Which foods are especially likely to cause GERD?

1. Chocolate & peppermint
2. Fatty meals
3. Alcohol

Mnemonic:
Think of someone eating a large crème de menthe sundae & getting heartburn –
That's mint, high-quality (fatty) ice cream, chocolate, and alcohol in the crème de menthe

When might you do 24-h esophageal pH monitoring?

To confirm GERD with an atypical presentation

Or

To assess how well medication is working

Esophageal biopsy provides some information in addition to the status of the epithelium. What other information does it give?

Allergic or infectious esophagitis can be identified

Is empiric proton pump inhibitor treatment as good for diagnosing GERD as EGD or 24-h monitoring?

No –
75 % sensitivity, but only 55 % specificity

(specific numbers not important – in other words, response doesn't tell you whether GERD was the cause)

**When should you definitely investigate GERD with endoscopy?
(3)**

Patient has:

1. **Weight loss**
2. **GI bleeding**
3. **Immunocompromise**

What is esophageal manometry useful for in patients who seem to have GERD?

r/o scleroderma
r/o achalasia

(It checks peristaltic motion and the lower esophageal sphincter tone)

Is dysphagia or odynophagia (difficulty or pain with swallowing) a sign that further investigation of GERD is needed?

Yes
(clinical evaluation is not sufficient)

If the GERD symptoms are continuously present for an extended time, or the symptoms don't respond to therapy, what should you do?

Confirm the diagnosis

Which patients are most likely to benefit from modification of diet, when GERD is suspected?

Patient is an infant

   Or

Milk or soy protein allergy may be present

What changes in the diet help infants with GERD?

(4)

1. Small volume, high-frequency feeds
2. Thickened feeds
3. Increased caloric content
4. Decreased crying time before feeding

Are obese patients at greater risk for GERD?

Yes –
Just a mechanical issue
(stomach is more compressed)

Infants with GERD have less difficulty with reflux if they are sleep prone. Should you recommend this?

No –
↑ incidence of SIDS

How does tobacco affect GERD?

Both ETOH & tobacco increase GERD

(passive smoke probably does, too, but data are less clear)

Does avoiding spicy foods help children with GERD?

**No –
But avoiding acidic ones will**

(tomatoes, chocolate, mints, some fruit)

Antacids have long-term use complications. What are they?

Aluminum & calcium
based → constipation

Magnesium based → diarrhea

(*Choose your poison, right?*)

What medications are considered "first line" for GERD?

Proton pump inhibitors

H$_2$ blockers (the "idine" family such as famotidine, ranitidine, etc.) may also be used, but are best for short term or supplemental acid control

When is it appropriate to use a longer course of proton pump inhibitor for reflux, such as 3–6 months?

Severe or erosive cases

How do proton pump inhibitors decrease acid secretion?

(Consider their name!)

They block the H/K ATPase proton pump

When are prokinetic agents useful for GERD?

When motility is the problem, such as with diabetic gastroparesis

Otherwise *not* useful!
(2009 FDA black box warning for metoclopramide)

How does erythromycin increase GI motility?

Motilin receptor agonist

(the other motility agents work differently)

What surgical options are available for reflux?

Fundoplication –
Refractory patients with serious sequelae

In simple terms, how does a fundoplication work?

Wraps the LES to create an artificial, but competent, sphincter

What is the rate of placebo response for GERD treatments?

25 %

Pretty good!

How long does it take for an H_2 blocker to provide some relief, if symptoms are present when it is taken?

About 30 min

Which reflux meds are most potent?

PPIs

(proton pump inhibitors)

What is the main feared complication of GERD?

Barrett's esophagus
(leading to adenocarcinoma)

What change constitutes "Barrett's esophagus?"

Metaplasia to columnar epithelium

(The esophagus should have squamous epithelium – like the inside of the cheek!)

Which patient group is at the greatest risk for adenocarcinoma of the esophagus?

White males
(incidence is increasing)

After Barrett's esophagus develops, will reflux treatment fix it?	No
How are esophageal strictures treated?	Dilation (by GI or surgery)
What is the main problem patients complain of with esophageal strictures?	Dysphagia & Food "sticking" at times
What is the special name for a stricture at the GE junction?	Schatzki's ring
If there are webs in the esophagus, what diagnoses should you think of? (2)	Diphtheria – *it could be the gray, adherent "pseudomembrane"* Or Plummer–Vinson syndrome – *glossitis (inflamed tongue), iron-deficiency anemia, and esophageal webs*
If a patient vomits blood (hematemesis), where is the bleeding coming from, anatomically speaking?	**Proximal to the "ligament of Treitz"** **(another way of saying upper GI bleed)**
If esophagitis is *not* due to infection or reflux, what other treatable cause might be found?	Eosinophilic (allergic) esophagitis
Why is it important to correctly identify eosinophilic esophagitis?	It is treatable (avoid allergen & give inhaled steroids) & It will not respond to treatments for other types of esophagitis
Painful swallowing, and retrosternal chest pain, especially in an immunocompromised patient, is likely to be what diagnosis?	Esophagitis (infective)

What organisms should you think of with infectious esophagitis?
(4)

- **Candida**
- **Herpes simplex or zoster**
- **CMV**
- **HIV**

Occasionally, increased pressure from vomiting, Valsalva, or CPR ruptures the esophagus.
What is this called?

Boerhaave tear

Is the Boerhaave tear of full thickness or just partial thickness?

Full thickness!

When Boerhaave's tear occurs in children & adults, where in the esophagus does it happen?

Left
Distal esophagus

Oddly enough, when Boerhaave's occurs in neonates, it occurs in a different spot. Where?

Right
Distal esophagus

Mnemonic:
Babies have extra stuff on the right, like the thymic shadow. This is on the right, too!

An esophageal tear can happen anytime we instrument the esophagus. What is the most common iatrogenic cause?

N-G tube placement

Other than pain, what do you expect to see on exam of someone with a tear in the esophagus?

Crepitus/air –
Usually subQ air in the neck,
or whichever part of the body
is the highest

Can esophageal full-thickness tears be treated conservatively, without surgery?

Generally, no –
Too much bad stuff can get into the mediastinum

What mediastinal signs would you look for on the chest X-ray, if esophageal rupture is suspected?

Wide mediastinum

&

Pneumomediastinum

What pulmonary findings are sometimes seen on chest X-ray with a Boerhaave's tear?

Pneumothorax

    &

Pleural effusion (usually left)

How could you radiologically confirm an esophageal rupture?

- Gastrografin esophagogram (it's water soluble, so not as bad as barium)

- CT scan

(Endoscopy is also sometimes used)

Why is a Mallory–Weiss tear so much less serious than Boerhaave's syndrome?

Mallory–Weiss is a <u>partial tear</u> – Boerhaave's is of full thickness

What usually happens to esophageal varices when a porto-systemic shunt is placed?

They usually involute (disappear)

What prophylactic treatment is helpful for patients with esophageal varices?

β-blockers

(sclerosing of esophageal varices *before* they bleed also reduces initial bleeds in kids, but the long-term benefit is not clear, and gastric venous issues may be increased)

In general, how are most foreign bodies managed?

They usually pass on their own

If the child eats a button battery, what should be done?

Remove it (usually endoscopically)

If a simple battery is eaten, when is it essential to remove it?

If it is impacted

Assuming that they don't pass right through, where do most objects get stuck in the digestive system? (5 spots)

In anatomic order:

1. **Cricopharyngeus muscle (upper esophageal sphincter)**

2. **Aortic arch**

3. **Lower esophageal sphincter**

4. **Pylorus**

5. **Ileocecal valve**

In addition to button batteries, what other objects need to be removed endoscopically?

Very sharp objects (such as razor blades or straight needles)

Should you use a gas-forming agent to build up the pressure to push a foreign body into the stomach?

**No –
The esophagus could rupture**

Why has papain (a meat tenderizer) fallen out of favor as a way to get rid of meat stuck in the esophagus?

What other meat is down there?
The esophagus itself (!) can be digested by it

What is the most effective way to manage something impacted in the esophagus?

Endoscopically

(remove it – usually by pushing it into the stomach)

What medical therapies can be tried for esophageal food impaction?

Glucagon

Or

**Nifedipine
(calcium channel blocker)**

What is the idea behind medical therapies for impacted esophageal items?

Relax the lower esophageal sphincter, so items can pass into the stomach

How should you verify that a swallowed foreign body is passing appropriately?
(2)

Have the caretakers watch for the object in the stool

&

**Serial X-rays
(make sure that it exits the stomach, make sure that it exits the colon)**

How can you tell whether a coin is in the esophagus or the trachea, based on the X-ray?

On an AP neck film:

- **The coin sits "flat" in the esophagus**

- **The coin is "on edge" if it is in the trachea**

Why do coins sit "on edge" in the neck if they are lodged in the trachea?

The tracheal cartilage is C-shaped, so it's open at the back. The coin fits best if it's stuck in that groove

If an object makes it into the stomach, is it likely to cause a problem?	No – Most things pass fine if they get into the stomach
When children ingest a foreign body, do they usually have symptoms from it?	No
As non-surgeons, what is the pediatrician's main role in managing pyloric stenosis?	**Correct fluids & electrolytes**
What metabolic derangement of pH will many pyloric stenosis babies have?	**Metabolic alkalosis** **(Remember, they are vomiting out acid, so they should get alkalotic)**
What post-op complication is especially likely in infants with metabolic alkalosis?	**Apnea!!!** (After all, one response to metabolic alkalosis is hypoventilation to increase acid content …)
What criteria must be met to diagnose pyloric stenosis?	Length >14 mm Thickness >4 mm (4 & 14)
What type of liquid ingestion is <u>most dangerous</u>?	**A base –** Liquefactive necrosis (it "melts" the tissue like a bad horror movie)
What should you do, other than ABC's, for someone who has ingested a base?	Arrange for endoscopy (Diluting with milk or water could be the right answer on an exam, if there aren't any better choices)
What must you <u>not</u> do for a patient who has ingested a base?	• **No lavage (more damage)** • **No charcoal (scope can't see a thing!)**
What are the main complications of eating a base (or a very bad acid)? **(4)**	1. **Perforation** 2. **Mediastinitis** 3. **Esophagitis** 4. **Strictures (later)**

Are steroids useful for patients who drank a base?

Sometimes –
With bad damage, stricture formation is reduced (not used routinely, though)

What two disorders produce gastric outlet obstruction in newborns?
(2)

Pyloric atresia

&

Antral webs

What prenatal conditions do babies with gastric outlet obstruction often develop?

Small for gestational age

&

Polyhydramnios

What scary complication can sometimes develop in infants with gastric outlet obstruction, even in the first 12 h of life?

Stomach rupture!

(antral webs are not as much of a problem)

How are antral webs and pyloric atresia treated?

NG tube
IV fluids
Surgical repair

What radiological findings confirm that your patient has gastric outlet obstruction?
(2)

Dilated stomach on X-ray

&

"Pyloric dimple" on an upper GI series confirms the diagnosis

What is "gastric duplication?"

Tubular or cystic structures found in the stomach wall

(they are leftovers from early development)

It's not two stomachs!

In what part of the stomach are gastric duplications usually found?

Greater curvature
(they are not open to the lumen)

What problems do gastric duplications cause?

- **Gastric outlet obstruction**
- **Gastric bleeding/ulceration**

How are gastric duplications diagnosed?

CT scan with contrast is best –
Upper GI series or US will also sometimes identify them

If a gastric duplication is symptomatic, how is it treated?	Surgery
In addition to the stomach, where else in the gut are "duplications" sometimes found?	Ileum (it is theoretically possible for them to occur anywhere in the gut)
When gut duplication occurs, what mucosal problem is often found in the duplication?	Ectopic mucosa (often gastric)
Which portion of the intestine is most often atretic?	Duodenum (as in, duodenal atresia)
Which type of atresia sometimes causes jaundice?	Duodenal (33 % of duodenal atresia patients will develop jaundice – Only happens if the bile outlet is blocked)
If you have a patient with duodenal atresia, what other abnormalities should you check for?	1. Gut stuff – malrotation, other atresias, anorectal problems 2. Down syndrome 3. Cardiac problems
Any type of bowel atresia will have what findings on X-ray?	• Air-filled, distended bowel *above* the atresia • Lack of bowel air below
What is the special radiological finding that goes with duodenal atresia?	**"Double-bubble" sign – Stomach bubble is seen, then a prominent duodenal bubble**
Are patients with any form of bowel atresia likely to be born pre-term, term, or postterm?	Preterm
With jejunal or ileal atresia, is the baby likely to pass meconium?	No – 75 % don't
What is gastric volvulus?	Rotation of the stomach – Either up & down or side to side (ouch!)
How is gastric volvulus treated?	**Surgically – Need to untwist and fix it in place (or it may happen again)**

How do you diagnose gastric volvulus?
(patient presentation)
(physical exam tipoff)
(radiological findings)

- Patient has severe pain and intractable vomiting
- NG won't pass
- Distended and sometimes twisted stomach on X-ray with *"beaking"* *at ends*

("beaking" means it narrows down at the end, like a beak)

If an infant has meconium ileus, what is the probability that he/she has CF?

90 %

Is meconium ileus a common problem for CF patients?

Not really –
10 % of CF patients have it

(If they have it, they're likely to have CF – but most CF patients don't have it)

How can you diagnose meconium peritonitis?

<u>Peritoneal calcifications</u> **with multiple air/fluid levels**

In meconium ileus, where is the majority of the meconium stuck?

Last 20–30 cm of the distal ileum

What does "complicated" meconium ileus mean?

There is a structural abnormality involved (such as volvulus or perforation)

How does meconium ileus look different from meconium peritonitis on X-ray?

Meconium ileus – ground glass look in the RLQ

Meconium peritonitis – patchy calcifications, especially in the flanks

Are enemas a good way to handle meconium ileus?

Gastrografin® enemas are acceptable – Risks are perforation & dehydration (due to the content of enema)

If the meconium ileus case is complicated, due to either bowel abnormalities or difficulties with enema therapy, how is it then treated?

Surgically

Why does malrotation happen?

The intestine fails to complete its embryological rotation

What is the main risk with malrotation?

Twisting the SMA (superior mesenteric artery) – Produces lots of bowel death!

When is malrotation most likely to present?

First year of life

(but can present years later)

When malrotation presents in the older child, what is its typical presentation?

Intermittent abdominal pain ± bilious emesis

One radiological finding that suggests your patient may have malrotation is finding a particular part of the gut in an unusual location. Which part of the gut is it?

Cecum
(various locations are possible)

What is the best way to diagnose malrotation in a newborn?

Upper GI

Are infants with atresia typical born full term or preterm?

Preterm

Can Hirschsprung's disease cause obstruction in the small intestine?

Yes –
But *only if* it extends to the terminal ileum (rare)

Patchy calcifications in the flanks on abdominal X-ray suggest what diagnosis?

Meconium *peritonitis*

Ground glass appearance in the right lower quadrant on X-ray of an infant suggests what diagnosis?

Meconium *ileus*

Where is it easiest to see free abdominal air on X-ray?

Under the diaphragm – Especially on the liver side!!!

(*Chest X-ray is best!*)

What complications are seen with the use of enemas in small children?

Perforation

&

Dehydration

What complications are seen with the use of gastrografin in kids?	Dehydration & Shock (due to volume loss)
If meconium ileus is treated with water-soluble enemas, how likely is it to work?	50 %
If a meconium ileus patient does not respond to medical interventions, and the patient does not have volvulus, atresia, or a perforation, what may be needed?	Surgery – End-to-end reanastomosis (colostomy is not normally needed)
When malrotation is corrected surgically, is the orientation of the gut changed?	No – The bands that the gut is "stuck on" are cut, but the gut will remain malrotated for life (Normal anatomical arrangement is not the goal – just prevention of future problems)
In Hirschsprung's, which nerve plexus is missing?	They both are (Meissner's & Auerbach's)
Hirschsprung's is associated with which congenital syndromes (mainly)? (5)	1. *Down* 2. *Waardenburg's (white forelock of hair)* 3. Cartilage hair 4. Ondine's curse (hypoventilation) 5. Smith–Lemli–Opitz (SLO) *The first two are most important*!
How common is it for Hirschsprung's babies to pass meconium in the first 24 h?	**Uncommon – Only about 6 % do**
When are adhesions most likely to cause problems, in relation to the timing of the surgery?	**Second week post-op**
If the problem is abdominal adhesions, how will the bowel sounds be described?	**"Hyperactive" (as with any obstruction)**

Ulcers are most likely to develop in the stomach as a result of NSAID use when what two medication situations occur?

Multiple- or high-dose NSAIDs are used

Or

Steroids are also given

How do infants & toddlers with peptic ulcer disease present?
(3)

1. Recurrent vomiting
2. GI hemorrhage
3. Slow growth

How do school-aged children with peptic ulcer disease present?

Same as adults –
Epigastric pain & GI bleeding

Periumbilical pain after eating is the usual presentation of peptic ulcer disease in which age group?

Preschoolers

Recurrent vomiting and GI bleed is the way gastric ulcers usually present in which age group?

Infants/toddlers

Preschool children with gastric ulcers usually have what complaint?

Periumbilical pain *after eating*

What is the gold standard for diagnosing ulcer disease?

Upper endoscopy

Are barium studies a good way to diagnose peptic ulcer disease?

Yes

(not as good for small mucosal lesions, though)

Why do NSAIDs increase the risk of peptic ulcer disease?

They inhibit prostaglandin synthesis – That decreases the amount of protective mucous the gut makes

When is a peptic ulcer considered to be "refractory" to treatment?

Not healed after 12 weeks of acid suppression

If a patient develops refractory peptic ulcers, what should you consider as possible causes to investigate?
(4)

1. *H. pylori*
2. NSAIDs
3. Cancer (presenting as an ulcer)
4. Hypersecretory state (such as Zollinger–Ellison)

What oncological disorder is associated with *H. pylori* infection?	MALT lymphoma
What kind of a lymphoma *is* MALT?	Low grade B cell *(frequently confused info – the T on MALT does not mean that it's a T cell tumor)*
What is the best way to treat MALT?	Treat the *H. pylori* – It will often regress on its own *(takes about 1.5 years to go away, though!!!)*
What is "special" about the way MALT lymphoma spreads? If you are treating MALT, and waiting for it to regress, what will you need to do while you wait?	It stays in the mucosa and submucosa only Periodic endoscopy to monitor it
Should all patients with suspected peptic ulcer disease be tested for *H. pylori*?	No – Only those with documented ulcers or MALT
H. pylori is most likely to be resistant to what commonly used medication?	Metronidazole – 40 %!
How long should you give antibiotics to get rid of *H. pylori*?	1–2 weeks (triple antibiotics)
What is a good first-line regimen for treatment of *H. pylori*?	Amoxicillin Clarithromycin PPI (such as omeprazole)
What is the triad of Zollinger–Ellison syndrome?	1. Chronic peptic ulcer disease 2. Secretory diarrhea 3. Esophageal injury (due to acid)
How common is celiac disease, also known as celiac sprue?	Common (1 per 200 or so in the US and European population)

Which body cells cause celiac disease?

T cells

(immune response to gluten)

In addition to antigliadin and antiendomysial antibody, what other blood test is a marker for celiac disease?

Anti-TTG

(TTG = Tissue transglutaminase)

What supplements will celiac disease patients need while they are recovering?
(2 sets)

- Vitamin D & calcium (can't digest milk yet)
- Iron & folate (damage to small bowel makes it harder to get enough)

If celiac patients have a relapse (of diarrhea), what is the most common reason for it?

Failure to follow the diet
(of course!)

Is celiac disease associated with any oncology diseases? If so, what type(s)?

Yes –
MALT & upper GI cancers

What causes "tropical" sprue?

Chronic gut contamination by toxigenic coliform bacteria

(the cause isn't completely clear, but that's what we think causes it)

In what part(s) of the world is tropical sprue seen?

The *tropics*
(for once the name fits!)

What are the symptoms of tropical sprue?
(4)

Water diarrhea
Cramping
Gas (flatulence)
Anorexia

Tropical sprue patients might have low levels of which nutrients?

B12 & folate

How is tropical sprue treated?

Tetracycline for up to 6 months

&

B12/folate supplements

Short bowel syndrome patients are at higher risk for which types of stones?
(2)

Gallstones

&

Calcium oxalate renal stones

(calcium oxalate stone formation seems to increase in most malabsorptive states)

Bacterial overgrowth in the small bowel is associated with malabsorption of what types of nutrients?

All types!

How is bacterial overgrowth syndrome treated?

7–10 days of antibiotics

What is "protein-losing enteropathy?"

When <u>plasma</u> proteins are dumped into the gut

(This happens normally, but to a very small extent)

In what two general situations will protein-losing enteropathy develop?

Too much backpressure (CHF, blocked gut lymphatics, etc.)

Or

Damaged enterocytes
(gut mucosa is damaged)

Lack of which fat-soluble vitamin can cause neurological disease?

Vitamin E

What group of disorders is treated by giving only fructose sugars and avoiding glucose–galactose?

SGLT1 gene defects

(SGLT = sodium–glucose co-transport gene)

How do patients with glucose–galactose malabsorption present?

- Osmotic diarrhea (if they eat glucose or lactose)
- Dehydration (and secondary acidosis)

What unusual urine finding will glucose–galactose malabsorption patients have?

Glucosuria *regardless of blood sugar level*

If you test a glucose–galactose malabsorption patient's stool for reducing substances, what will you find?

It will be <u>positive</u>

(there are carbs in the urine – reducing substances are carbs)

What is the gene defect that causes glucose–galactose malabsorption?

SGLT1

(sodium–glucose co-transporter gene)

If the SGLT1 gene is defective, which cells will have difficulty transporting glucose & galactose?

Gut & renal cells

How is glucose–galactose malabsorption syndrome transmitted?	Autosomal recessive
If you do a biopsy on a patient with glucose–galactose malabsorption, will the villi be normal?	<u>Yes</u>
If a glucose–galactose malabsorption patient takes the hydrogen breath test, what will it show?	It will be positive (because there are extra sugars in the gut)
What is the *only sugar* a SGLT1 defect patient can absorb?	Fructose
What is the treatment for glucose–galactose malabsorption?	Give fructose & Avoid glucose/galactose
Absent deep tendon reflexes (DTRs) due to peripheral neuropathy can result from too little vitamin _____?	E
Acanthocytes on the peripheral blood smear is a buzzword for what genetic disorder? (*Very popular board question*)	**Abetalipoproteinemia**
What's an acanthocyte?	**RBCs that are spiky** (they have little spicules sticking out from their membranes)
What is the underlying problem in abetalipoproteinemia?	Congenital absence of apoB (B-lipoprotein cannot be made)
What is the importance of a child not being able to make B-lipoprotein?	**Chylomicrons (for fat transport) cannot be made**
What is the main nutritional consequence of abetalipoproteinemia?	**Severe congenital fat malabsorption**

How is abetalipoproteinemia treated?	• **Give fat-soluble vitamins** • *Give medium-chain* **fatty acids** • *Avoid long-chain* **fatty acids** **(otherwise just supportive care)**
How is abetalipoproteinemia inherited?	**Autosomal recessive**
What will you notice about the belly on physical exam of an abetalipoproteinemia infant?	Baby with big belly (distended abdomen) – Due to big stool volume
What is the usual description of an abetalipoproteinemia baby's stool?	Bulky & pale (all that extra fat in it)
What is the typical neurological finding for an abetalipoproteinemia baby?	DTRs are missing (*Due to vitamin E deficiency*)
Do abetalipoproteinemia babies grow normally?	No – FTT
So how do abetalipoproteinemia children present?	• Steatorrhea & distended belly • FTT • ↓ DTRs
How is "homozygous hypobetalipoproteinemia" different from abetalipoproteinemia? (3 ways)	• Dominant disorder • Parents have low levels of LDL • Small vacuoles are seen in the gut cells (large ones are seen in abetalipoproteinemia)
Is the *presentation* of infants with homozygous hypobetalipoproteinemia different from abetalipoproteinemia?	**No** **(the effect is the same)**
Over time, abetalipoproteinemia (and homozygous hypobetalipoproteinemia) patients develop what two important complications?	**Retinitis pigmentosa** **&** **Neurological problems** (ataxia & nystagmus due to lack of fat-soluble vitamins)

If chylomicrons are made, but cannot be expelled (exocytosed), the effect is similar to having no chylomicrons. Which disorder has this problem?

Anderson disease
Aka "chylomicron retention disease"

How is chylomicron retention disease different from abetalipoproteinemia?

- More diarrhea
- *Rare* *acanthocytes*
- *No severe neurological problems*
- No retinitis pigmentosa

What congenital cause of diarrhea involves an abnormal Cl/HCO$_3$ transporter?

Chloride-losing diarrhea

(autosomal recessive disorder)

How is chloride-losing diarrhea treated?

IV & oral electrolyte correction

(good prognosis)

How do chloride-losing diarrhea patients present at birth?

Severe, watery diarrhea
(*right at birth!*)

What prenatal abnormality is usually noted in chloride-losing diarrhea patients?

Polyhydramnios

(makes sense – a lot of excess fluid is produced)

How could an infant be B12 deficient due to inadequate intake?

(*popular question item*)

Vegan mother exclusively breast feeding

(vegan means does not eat eggs or milk products)

What unusual causes of congenital B12 problems are there?
(2)

Transcobalamine II deficiency (transport protein not available)

&

Imerslund syndrome
(ileum unable to absorb B12)

How can B12 deficiency be treated, if the patient has congenital malabsorption of B12?

IM injections

Or

Intranasal B12

Which patients are not candidates for intranasal B12 treatment?

Anemic patients –
The level needs to rise quickly & surely, so IM is better

What commonly used GI medication class can contribute to B12 deficiency?	**Gastric acid blocker** (*acid frees the B12 from food*)
In congenital chloride diarrhea, is the stool likely to have an acid or an alkalotic pH?	**Acid** **(the bicarb is being retained by the body to an unusually high degree)**
What is the pH of the patient likely to be in congenital chloride diarrhea?	**Alkalotic –** **Too much bicarb is retained** (*but normal or acidotic is also possible if the patient becomes very dehydrated & tissues are hypoperfused*)
If a patient has congenital diarrhea, and the stool is *not high in chloride*, what other congenital diarrhea should you consider?	Congenital sodium diarrhea (Na–H exchanger defect)
Other than dehydration, does congenital sodium diarrhea cause the patient problems?	No – Just rehydrate orally
What is the most common cause of congenital diarrhea? (*Very popular item!*)	**Congenital microvillus disease**
How is congenital microvillus inclusion disease inherited?	Recessive
What is the mortality rate for congenital microvillus disease?	BAD – 80 %
What do the "inclusions" refer to, in congenital microvillus inclusion disease?	**Microvilli sitting within the apical membrane** **(can be seen when you look with an electron microscope)**
How do congenital microvillus inclusion disease patients present?	**Malabsorption of everything** **&** **Severe watery diarrhea** (makes sense – absorptive surface is missing)

How can congenital microvillus inclusion disease be treated?	Total parenteral nutrition Or Small bowel transplant
If a newborn has low calcium and low magnesium, what diagnosis should you consider?	Primary hypomagnesemia
What is the main danger of hypomagnesemia?	Tetany (due to the accompanying hypocalcemia)
Is there a congenital form of rickets?	Yes (autosomal recessive)
Defective copper absorption leads to what syndrome?	**Menkes ("kinky hair") syndrome**
How is Menkes kinky hair syndrome inherited?	**Recessive**
On labs, how is Menkes syndrome like Wilson disease?	**Both have <u>low</u> serum ceruloplasmin levels**
How is Menkes syndrome treated?	**Parenteral copper**
In addition to affecting the hair, low serum copper levels lead to what other problem(s)? **(3)**	1. **Fractures** 2. **Bad vascular disease** 3. **Cerebellar degeneration**
What causes the problems in Wilson disease?	**Too much copper in the tissues**
Which organs are affected in Wilson disease?	**Liver** **&** **Brain** **(neurological & psychiatric changes)**
If a Wilson disease patient develops psychiatric symptoms, at what age will those symptoms usually present?	**School age or adolescence**

Generally, circulating copper levels are *low* in Wilson disease. At what point in the disease are they often high?

Early in the disease
(with accompanying liver failure)

What is the expected lab pattern for copper labs in Wilson disease?

Ceruloplasmin – LOW

What is the famous eye finding in Wilson disease?

Kayser–Fleischer ring

What does the famous eye finding of Wilson disease look like?

A milky ring just inside the margin of the cornea

(it's copper in the cornea)

Is Wilson disease treatable?

**Yes –
Chelate the copper** &
Low-copper diet

(and screen other family members)

Will treating Wilson disease improve neurological problems that have already developed?

Yes

Unexplained liver disease, with neurological problems and psychiatric changes in a school-aged child should make you consider what diagnosis?

Wilson disease

(Frequently tested item!)

What is the gold standard for diagnosing Wilson disease?

Liver biopsy

In addition to the water supply, what other sources of dietary copper will Wilson patients need to avoid?

Shellfish
Liver
Nuts
Chocolate

Mnemonic:
Think of a really rich meal with most people's favorite foods – lobster, chocolate, macadamia nuts – all of these are high in copper (+ liver, of course)

What is neonatal hemochromatosis?	Elevated iron due to bad liver damage before birth (iron is deposited both in the liver & in extrahepatic sites)
Is neonatal hemochromatosis caused by the same genetic problem that causes most hereditary hemochromatosis?	No – The cause is unclear, & there may be several (maternal alloimmunity, mitochondrial disorder, & transplacental infective cause are all possibilities)
Which gene is the most common cause of hereditary hemochromatosis?	Mutation of the HFE gene (variable penetrance)
Does hereditary hemochromatosis require treatment during the pediatric years?	Usually not (may begin in adolescence)
How many types of progressive familial intrahepatic cholestasis (PFIC) are there?	Three
What is the main characteristic of the PFIC disorders?	Bad cholestasis and pruritus
Which of the three PFIC disorders is the worst?	PFIC 1 (Diarrhea, fat malabsorption, pancreatitis, early cirrhosis)
How is PFIC 3 different from the other two?	GGT is high (it is normal for the other two) & It presents later
How do PFIC 1 patients present?	• Early (3–6 months old) • Intense itching & high conjugated bili • Normal GGT
What in the world is Aagenaes syndrome?	Spontaneously resolving cholestasis & lymphedema in Norwegian newborns

Ileal absorption of bile acids depends on what type of transporter?

Sodium-dependent transplant

If bile acid transport is defective, what problems develop?
(4)

1. Diarrhea
2. Steatorrhea
3. Low cholesterol
4. Low fat-soluble vitamin levels

Zinc malabsorption leads to what problem?

Acrodermatitis enteropathica

What is the main symptom or sign of zinc deficiency?

Rash at mucocutaneous junction

(also hair loss & extremity rashes)

What readily available lab test will be low if the zinc level is low?

Alkaline phosphatase

In low-zinc states, what will you see in intestinal Paneth cells?

Inclusions
(they disappear after treatment)

Acrodermatitis enteropathica is due to what deficiency?

Low zinc *due to zinc malabsorption*

(*Very common question!*)

When will infants with acrodermatitis enteropathica first develop symptoms?

About 1 month after birth

Or

1 month after discontinuing breast feeding

How is acrodermatitis enteropathica treated?

Oral elemental zinc

Cholestyramine binds bile salts but also binds which important element?

Calcium

(can result in hypocalcemia)

What commonly used seizure medication interferes with calcium absorption, sometimes leading to rickets?

Phenytoin

(Dilantin®)

A vignette of a child who moves slowly, a little hunched over, who is also limping on the right side may indicate what surgical diagnosis?

Appendicitis

A history of painless rectal bleeding in a child or a young adult with a family history of colectomy suggests what diagnosis? | Familial adenomatous Polyposis coli

If an intussusception is jejuno-jejunal, what unusual cause for a lead point should you consider? | Polyp in a patient with Peutz–Jeghers

Are Peutz–Jeghers patients at increased risk for GI cancers? | **No –** **They are at increased risk for cancer _outside_ the GI tract**

Is Peutz–Jeghers usually inherited, or does it usually come from a new mutation? | 50/50

How can you recognize a Peutz–Jeghers patient? | Freckling of lips/gums, hands, & genitals

What is abnormal about the gut in Peutz–Jeghers patients? | There are hamartomas & polyps

Are hemangiomas in the gut a problem? | Sometimes – They can bleed profusely and sometimes cause intussusception or obstruction

(otherwise benign)

What benign cause of GI pain & bleeding is sometimes treated with steroids? | Nodular lymphoid hyperplasia (NLH)

Pancreatic dysfunction in a patient with _cyclic neutropenia_ & anemia = | **Shwachman–Diamond syndrome**

CT & MRI will both show what finding in the pancreas of Shwachman–Diamond patients? | Fatty appearance, with little fibrosis

Which aspects of the pancreas are _normal_ in Shwachman–Diamond syndrome?

(2 components) | Ducts

&

Islet cells

Shwachman–Diamond syndrome patients present similarly to what common recessive disorder in the white European population?	CF (but the sweat test is <u>normal</u> for S-D patients)
Both Shwachman–Diamond & CF have short stature and FTT, along with pancreatic dysfunction. How is the S-D presentation different? (2 main aspects)	1. Recurrent pyogenic infections (neutrophil chemotaxis problem) 2. Anemia/thrombocytopenia are common for S-D
A pancreas with intact ducts, but lots of fatty replacement and little fibrosis, is characteristic of what disorder?	Shwachman–Diamond (+ *cyclic neutropenia*)
Pancreatic insufficiency, dwarfism, & missing permanent teeth should make you think of what syndrome?	Johanson–Blizzard Mnemonic: Think of a dwarf with a fat belly (can't absorb it) standing in a blizzard
Nesidioblastosis (new name: nonfamilial hyperinsulinemic hypoglycemia) requires the patient to undergo what surgery?	Pancreatectomy (to control low glucose)
What is the most common pancreatic disorder of childhood?	Acute pancreatitis (usually viral)
If the liver is no longer able to synthesize things like albumin & coagulation factors, how much of the liver is damaged/dead?	75 %
What endocrine problem should you rule out in an infant with neonatal cholestasis?	Hypothyroidism – Everything is slow, including the bile
What inherited disorder should you rule out in infants with neonatal cholestasis?	CF
Amino acid levels in the serum & urine, along with urine-reducing substances, allow you to evaluate for what general cause of neonatal cholestasis?	Metabolic liver disease

What level of conjugated circulating bilirubin (%) is always considered pathological?	>20 % (conjugated hyperbilirubinemia is always something to investigate, this cutoff just tells you when the number is high enough to consider it "conjugated hyperbilirubinemia")
If a neonate's bilirubin is <5 mg/dL, what level of conjugated bilirubin is considered pathological?	1.0 mg/dL
How common is biliary atresia?	1/15,000 live births
What does "triangular cord" refer to, when seen in an infant's abdomen?	A cone-shaped fibrotic mass near the liver – Goes with biliary atresia
What vascular system abnormalities are commonly seen in infants with biliary atresia?	Polysplenia (multiple spleens) & Vascular malformations
Why is a HIDA-type scan of the liver a somewhat limited test for diagnosing biliary atresia?	It is not very specific (will show uptake, but no excretion)
How is biliary atresia evaluated in *all* patients?	Exploratory laparotomy – Correct lesion if possible
If a particular patient's biliary atresia cannot be corrected, what is done for the patient?	Kasai (The Kasai procedure is a hepatoportoenterostomy)
On biopsy, what do you expect to see with biliary atresia? (4)	1. Bile duct proliferation 2. Fibrosis 3. Bile "plugs" 4. Edema, but lobular architecture is okay
If a patient has hepatitis, what do you expect to see on biopsy? (4)	1. Distorted architecture 2. Inflammatory cells 3. Normal, intact, bile ducts 4. Focal areas of necrosis

What is the point of giving phenobarbital to patients undergoing liver/biliary HIDA scanning?	It speeds up the excretion process (if there is no obstruction)
How is Crigler–Najjar type 1 different from C-N type 2?	Type 1 is more uncommon, usually fatal, and has no bili conjugation at all
What two options are available for treating Crigler–Najjar type 1?	Phototherapy & Liver transplant
Why do Crigler–Najjar type 1 children die?	Fatal kernicterus
How is Crigler–Najjar type 2 different from type 1?	Enzyme function is 10 % of normal, so kernicterus is rare
How is Crigler–Najjar II treated? (Type 2 = type II)	Phenobarbital induces greater enzyme activity, lowering bili to acceptable levels (but normally no treatment is needed)
Even in untreated type II Crigler–Najjar, is kernicterus a problem?	No – The enzyme activity is sufficient (except in rare cases in which the patient was stressed by fasting, general anesthesia, or illness)
Are LFTs elevated in Crigler–Najjar?	No
If a very jaundiced infant, without evidence of biliary obstruction, has *no bili* in the urine, what genetic disorder should you consider?	Crigler–Najjar type 1 – If no bili is conjugated, no urobilinogen is made!
In what age group(s) is Gilbert's syndrome usually diagnosed?	**Adolescence or adulthood**
How do Gilbert's syndrome patients present?	**Increased bili with stress, ETOH, low calories (a form of stress), etc.**
What is the underlying problem that creates Gilbert's syndrome?	**A 1/3 reduction in enzyme activity (the enzyme is UDP-glucuronosyltransferase)**

Crigler–Najjar types 1 & 2, and Gilbert's syndrome, all result from missing or decreased function of what enzyme?

UDP-glucuronosyltransferase

While disorders with decreased UDP-glucuronosyltransferase produce high unconjugated bili, Dubin–Johnson syndrome produces an increase in what sort of bilirubin?

Conjugated

Dark pigment in lysosomes **is classic for the histology of what GI disorder?**

Dubin–Johnson

(also causes a black liver on gross inspection)

Females with Dubin–Johnson should avoid what common medication?

Oral contraceptives

The gross appearance of the liver in Dubin–Johnson is _____?

Black!

Mnemonic:
Remember that they have dark pigment in their lysosomes – dark lysosomes/ dark liver

Which types of viral hepatitis are acquired through fecal-oral transmission?

A&E

A vaccine for hepatitis A is available. Which non-immunized patient groups most benefit from hepatitis A immunization?

- Travelers
- Those with severe liver impairment
- Men having sex with men

(Immunization is now recommended for all US children at one year old.)

If someone is exposed to hepatitis A, and he/she is not immune, is there anything you can do to prevent infection from developing?

Yes –
Give hepatitis A immunoglobulin

How successful is hepatitis A immunoglobulin for preventing infection?

Somewhat

When a case of hepatitis A occurs, who should routinely be given post-exposure prophylaxis?

Household and intimate contacts

Is hepatitis A immunoglobulin used in any other situation?

Yes –
Can also give it prophylactically, when exposure is anticipated

(e.g., for travelers who don't have time for the immunization to work)

Can hepatitis A be transmitted transplacentally?

No

Does hepatitis A exist in a carrier or a chronic state?

No – neither

Are hepatitis B viruses shed in breast milk?

Yes –
But in very low levels

Is it alright for a hepatitis B-positive mother to breast-feed her infant?

Yes

In chronic hepatitis B infection, how long should the surface antigen (HepBsAg) remain positive?

≥6 months

Which patients are most likely to develop chronic Hep B infection?

The youngest

(most likely if <1 year old)

What autoimmune/rheumatological disorder is highly associated with hepatitis B infection?

Polyarteritis nodosa

What is the main serological marker for hepatitis B replication & infectivity?

HBe Ag

(others are HBV DNA & HBV Pol)

What is the order of appearance for serological markers of hepatitis B infection?

Hep B surface <u>antigen</u>

Hep B core anti<u>body</u>

Hep B surface anti<u>body</u>

How long is the hepatitis B incubation period?

1–6 months

Hepatitis B vaccination requires how many injections and at what intervals?	• Three injections • 0, 1, & 6 months (there are multiple acceptable schedules)
If you find Hep B surface antigen in an asymptomatic patient, what should you do?	Just follow – Vaccine & Ig do not help if the patient is already infected
If you have just delivered a newborn to a Hep B-positive mother, what should you do?	Give Ig and vaccine – It may prevent infection
Titers of what in the blood indicate immunity to hepatitis B? (Due to either infection or immunization)	**Anti-HepBsAg antibody** **(Hepatitis B surface antigen *antibody*)**
How can you tell whether a patient is immune to Hep B due to immunization or prior infection?	If IgG antibody to Hep B *core antigen* is present, immunity is from prior infection
To recap, what is the importance of HepBe antigen & antibodies?	• **HepBe antigen indicates the level of liver inflammation and infectivity** • **The antibody appears several weeks after the antigen**
Can chronic viral hepatitis patients have normal ALT levels?	**Yes –** **Sometimes the value returns to normal for brief periods**
Not all Hep B carriers have the "chronic hepatitis B" type of infection. For those that do, what problems are they at risk for in adulthood? (2)	Cirrhosis & Hepatocellular cancer
After resolution of an acute Hep B infection, what should you check several months later? (2)	HBV DNA & HepB surface Ag (if they are not gone, your patient is in a carrier state)

Board exams are famous for asking about the "window period." What does the "window period" for Hep B infection refer to?

The time when HepBsAg and HepBsAb are undetectable

(the quantity of each is in balance, so they bind to each other, and can't be detected)

In the window period, how can you detect the presence of Hep B infection?

Anti-HepBc IgM

(IgM antibody to Hep B core antigen)

Which viral hepatidity can *only occur* in the presence of hepatitis B infection?

Hep D

Mnemonic:
"D" is "defective" – it needs B to help it

If a patient contracts hepatitis D while actively infected with hepatitis B, what is the usual course of the disease?

Severe

If hepatitis D is contracted *at the same time* as hepatitis B, does it make much difference to the course of the disease?

No

What does the "window period" for hepatitis B infection refer to?

The time when HepBsAg *and* HepBsAb are undetectable –
This happens because the amount of antigen and antibody are in perfect balance, so all of them are bound to each other

When viral hepatitis occurs as a noticeable epidemic (usually in developing countries), which type is usually responsible?

E

Mnemonic:
"E" is for "epidemic"

Which usually mild viral hepatitis is much more virulent in pregnancy women?

Hepatitis E

Mnemonic:
You know that "B" & "C" are bad to have ("bad cases"). "D" is "defective." By process of elimination, "E" is the one that is vicious for pregnant people

Most transfusion-associated hepatitis is what type?

Hepatitis C

How likely is a HepC infection to become chronic?

**Very likely
(roughly 80 %)**

Two to four months after an episode of hepatitis C, how can you check whether the infection has become chronic?	Do a PCR for HCV-RNA
What percentage of patients who contract HepC is aware of the infection?	25 %
What vasculitis is especially associated with Hep C (although it can also occur with Hep B)?	Mixed cryoglobulinemia – A small vessel vasculitis
How does mixed cryoglobulinemia present?	Palpable purpura or "crops" (groups) of purple papules
Which ethnic groups are usually able to process lactose easily throughout the life-span?	Northern & Central European ancestry
Infants should never be lactose deficient, unless the villi (brush border) have been damaged or they have which genetic disorder?	**Congenital lactase deficiency (makes sense)** *Autosomal recessive inheritance*
In which country or ethnic group is the inherited problem with lactose processing found most often?	Finland/Finnish people
What recessive disorder first becomes noticeable when sucrose is given to an older infant?	Sucrase-isomaltase deficiency
How is sucrase-isomaltase deficiency treated?	Oral "sacrosidase" replaces the enzyme
Celiac disease is 50 times more common in which patient population, compared to the general population?	**Down**
Autoimmune diseases and celiac disease often co-occur. Which two autoimmune disorders should make you screen for celiac disease, automatically?	Type I DM & IgA deficiency (selective deficiency)

Celiac disease patients are at risk for what annoying dermatologic condition?	Dermatitis herpetiformis
Very itchy bullous lesions on extensor surfaces and the scalp indicate what diagnosis?	Dermatitis herpetiformis *(Has no connection to herpes, by the way!)*
Whipple disease is rarely seen in kids. What is it, and how is it treated? **(*Very popular item*!)**	• **Gut infection with *T. whippelii*** • **Antibiotics ≥6 months**
What problems does Whipple disease cause?	Severe malabsorption + Rheumatological & neurological complaints
What is "typhlitis?"	**Inflammation of the cecum**
Which patients develop typhlitis?	**Immunocompromised – Especially leukemia patients**
Why is typhlitis important? **(2 reasons)**	1. **It presents very similarly to appendicitis** 2. **High risk of gangrene & perforation**
If a neutropenic patient develops typhlitis, what does this mean for their future?	The typhlitis is likely to recur in later periods of neutropenia
How is typhlitis treated?	Bowel rest & antibiotics
A 5-year-old child presents with painless rectal bleeding, noted only with bowel movements. There is no significant family history. What kind of polyp is likely to cause this?	A juvenile polyp
How are "juvenile polyps" different from "juvenile polyposis?"	1. **Less than five polyps** 2. **No family history of polyp syndromes** 3. **<u>Not</u> a cancer risk**

If you find a single polyp in a family member of someone who had juvenile polyposis, what diagnosis should you make?

Juvenile polyposis

How should a child with painless rectal bleeding be evaluated, in most cases?

Colonoscopy

(& biopsy any polyps found)

What is the most common malignant tumor of the small intestine in children?

Lymphoma (!)

Familial adenomatous polyposis syndromes are the result of what genetic mutation?

Chromosome 5q21–22

Mnemonic:
You'd have at least 5 polyps, so its found on 5q

What is the inheritance pattern for familial adenomatous polyposis syndrome?

Autosomal *dominant*
(with variable penetrance)

What proportion of familial adenomatous polyposis patients present without family history (new mutations)?

1/3

What is Gardner's syndrome?

Polyposis coli

  +

Extraintestinal tumors

How should Gardner's syndrome patients be managed?

- Screening colonoscopy beginning age 10 years

- Yearly colonoscopy

- Thyroid & upper GI screen (due to increased risk in those areas)

Hemihypertrophy & hamartomas (gut or elsewhere) = what diagnosis?

Proteus syndrome

(has nothing to do with the microbiology "proteus")

There is a group of very unusual disorders linked to dysfunction of the PTEN gene. Proteus syndrome is one of them. In general, what are the characteristics of these disorders? (Six characteristics – spells "MATCHS")

Macrocephaly
Autosomal dominant
Thyroid disease
Cancer
Hamartomas
Skin abnormalities

Mnemonic:
Protean means "many." You will need some "matchs" that illuminate the cause of many different abnormalities

What does the PTEN gene do?

Regulates tyrosine phosphatase

How can you remember that PTEN problems cause proteus and related disorders?

The patients have "protean" (many) problems – you could have ten problems in one patient!

PTEN = Proteus patient with TEN problems

What is gastroschisis?

A separation in the abdominal wall

(the two sides didn't fuse lengthwise)

Where on the belly will you find the defect in gastroschisis?

Lateral

Do solid organs come through a gastroschisis or only intestines?

Only intestine, usually

Will the bowel projecting through a gastroschisis have a peritoneal covering?

No –
Peritoneum formation was also disrupted!

How is gastroschisis managed?

SURGERY ASAP!

Do gastroschisis patients usually have associated anomalies?

No

How is an omphalocele different from gastroschisis?
             (4 differences)

- **Solid organs are often involved**

- ***It is covered by peritoneum***

- **Associated abnormalities are common**

- **Location is periumbilical**

How is an omphalocele different from an umbilical hernia?

Umbilical hernias are smaller (<4 cm) & *do not involve solid organs*

What is the initial management of either omphalocele or gastroschisis?

Keep it wet & warm!

- **Saline-soaked gauze** (wet)
- **Plastic wrap** (warm & retains moisture)
- **Make sure that the gut isn't twisted** (perfusion keeps it warm)

Is it alright to delay closure of an omphalocele?

Yes

Is it alright to delay closure of a gastroschisis?

**No
(it's not covered)**

What is pseudo-Hirschsprung's disease?

A collection of disorders with either nerve problems or muscle problems in the gut

What is "hypoganglionosis" of the gut, and how does it present?

- Congenital or acquired decrease in the number of gut neurons
- Constipation (severe & chronic)

How is intestinal neuronal dysplasia diagnosed?

Full-thickness biopsy (shows giant ganglia & hyperganglionosis)

Macrocytic anemia & pancreatic exocrine dysfunction (± other hematologic abnormalities) is likely to be what diagnosis?

"Pearson pancreatic & bone marrow syndrome"
(aka Pearson syndrome)

What is the initial radiological test of choice for evaluating the pancreas?

Ultrasound

In an adolescent patient with acute pancreatitis, what etiology should you consider?

ETOH

Patients on what class of drugs are at increased risk for pancreatitis?

**Antiretroviral for HIV
(such as ddI)**

A severe form of acute pancreatitis is frequently presented on the boards. What is it?

Acute hemorrhagic pancreatitis

Why is acute hemorrhagic pancreatitis important (since it's not very common)?

50 % mortality

What two abdominal signs are often given in the vignette for acute hemorrhagic pancreatitis (due to the bleeding from the pancreas)?

Cullen's sign – bluish discoloration at the umbilicus (due to accumulated blood)

Grey–Turner – same on the flanks

What is the drug of choice for pain control in pancreatitis?

Meperidine (Demerol®)

(Some sources now also recommend morphine, but this is a long-standing area of debate. There is evidence that morphine can cause spasm of the sphincter of Oddi, which may not be ideal for pancreatitis patients.)

Which lab test is most reliable for diagnosing pancreatitis?

Lipase

How is pancreatitis treated?
        (3 main components)

- **Bowel rest**
- **Pain control**
- **Maintain hydration/electrolytes**

Most patients with congenital hepatic fibrosis also have what congenital renal disorder?

Polycystic kidney disease (recessive type)

Why does congenital hepatic fibrosis cause problems?
                (2)

The deranged architecture sometimes leads to portal hypertension

&

Risk of cholangitis

How is congenital hepatic fibrosis diagnosed?

Biopsy

What is Caroli disease?

Congenital dilatation of the large intrahepatic bile ducts

If a patient has both Caroli disease (dilated large ducts) and congenital hepatic fibrosis, what is that called?

Caroli syndrome

How do Caroli disease/syndrome patients present?

Recurrent cholangitis & abscesses
beginning in adolescence or adulthood

Does Caroli disease/syndrome always affect the entire liver?

No –
Sometimes it is limited to one area

Children with Alagille syndrome have what characteristic facies?

Elvin

(Elvin means "like an elf." Think of Liv Tyler's face – she played the elf princess in the Hobbit series)

What is the main hallmark of Alagille syndrome?

Neonatal cholestasis with a "paucity" of small ducts

What funny bone findings point you toward a diagnosis of Alagille syndrome?

Butterfly vertebrae

&

Abnormal radius/ulna

What is the main abnormality that causes Alagille syndrome patients problems?

Pulmonary artery stenosis

What is the prognosis for Alagille patients?

Not terrible –
25 % die due to associated problems

What is the usual course for liver function in Alagille patients?

Most develop normal function over the first year of life

Is the Kasai procedure a good idea for Alagille syndrome kids?

No

Alagille syndrome patients are at unusually high risk for bleeding from what type of trauma?

Head trauma –
Reason unknown

(still at risk even if liver function is normal)

How is Alagille syndrome inherited?

Autosomal dominant
(variable penetrance)

Just to be sure you remember, what is the underlying problem in Dubin–Johnson syndrome?

Deficiency of the transporter
(for conjugated bili)

In most cases, how is drug toxicity affecting the liver treated?	Supportive care
Which anesthetic agent is known for sometimes inducing liver damage?	**Halothane**
Which common seizure medication is known for sometimes causing liver toxicity?	**Phenytoin**
Which IBD medication is known for sometimes causing liver toxicity?	**Sulfasalazine** **(methotrexate & 6-MP can also do it)**
What is the best known medication for inducing liver toxicity?	**Acetaminophen**
Acetaminophen has a particular antidote. What is it?	**_N_-acetylcysteine** **(aka NAC or mucomyst)**
Why is NAC helpful in Tylenol® overdose?	**It replenishes glutathione – the liver is then able to process the Tylenol® without making toxins**
Children rarely develop cholecystitis. When are they at greatest risk, though?	Following burn, trauma, or life-threatening illness (usually _acalculous_ cholecystitis – meaning no stones)
What is "hydrops" of the gall bladder?	Dilation/enlargement of the gall bladder for no apparent reason!
Do patients have any symptoms with hydrops of the gall bladder?	Yes – Fever, vomiting, jaundice, & RUQ pain are common!
Which patients are at risk to develop hydrops of the gall bladder due to their nutritional status?	Fasting patients & TPN patients
Which three rheumatological or autoimmune conditions put pediatric patients at risk to develop hydrops of the gall bladder?	HSP (Henoch–Schönlein purpura), Kawasaki disease, & Strep pharyngitis

How is gall bladder hydrops treated?

Supportive care (and resolve the underlying condition)

A very young infant with hepato-splenomegaly, multinucleated giant cells on liver biopsy, and no apparent infectious or metabolic cause, has what diagnosis?

Idiopathic neonatal hepatitis

(aka giant cell hepatitis)

What is the usual course for infants with idiopathic neonatal hepatitis?

75 % resolve spontaneously – The remainder develop cirrhosis

An adolescent with acne is being treated with doxycycline. He or she comes in with chest pain. What is the diagnosis?

(Popular item!)

Pill-induced esophagitis (pill sticks to esophagus & dissolves there, irritating the tissue)

How long does pill-induced esophagitis take to resolve?

About 2 weeks

If a child eats a caustic substance, what procedure must be done to evaluate the damage?

Endoscopy

When is the best time to perform the endoscopy to evaluate the upper gut, after ingestion of a caustic agent?

12–24 h after (damage cannot be fully assessed until at least 12 h have passed)

Which pills are most likely to cause pill-induced esophagitis?

Tetracyclines
Slow-release K
NSAIDs

Should you give a "neutralizing agent," like water or milk, if a caustic has been ingested?

No –
Not even water
(it may trigger vomiting and exothermic reactions)

Esophageal perforation is most likely in pediatric patients with which baseline disorders?

Ehlers–Danlos

&

Marfan's

(makes sense – their tissues aren't held together as well as usual – *can even happen spontaneously!*)

Along with chest & upper back pain, and subcutaneous emphysema, what unexpected findings often accompany esophageal perforation?
(2)

Fever (due to general inflammatory reaction)

&

Hypotension
(probably vagal)

If you suspect esophageal perforation, what studies should you use to confirm it?

Plain X-ray,
Then X-ray with a small amount of water-soluble contrast

(CT will also show it)

Can barium be used if esophageal perforation is suspected?

Yes –
If the water-soluble contrast study was not conclusive

Is achalasia a motor problem or an anatomic one?

Motor

So what exactly *is* achalasia?

Difficulty swallowing due to a disorder of esophageal motility

What is dysphagia?

Difficulty swallowing for <u>any</u> reason

What are the two causes of dysphagia (general categories)?

Motor (achalasia)

&

Mechanical or anatomic (strictures, diverticula, webs)

If achalasia presents in childhood, how old are the children likely to be?

About 10 years

Why do achalasia patients have difficulty swallowing?

The LES doesn't relax normally

(decreased ganglion cells in the esophagus)

If achalasia presents in a very young child, what are you likely to be dealing with?

A genetic syndrome

(a rare one, such as "Allgrove" syndrome)

What is "cyclic vomiting?"

Spells of very frequent vomiting with no apparent cause

Who is likely to develop cyclic vomiting?

6–7-year-old girls, with a strong family history of migraine

What is marasmus?

Calorie malnutrition

(skinny kids, like the pictures of people from the concentration camps)

Protein malnutrition is also known as _____?

Kwashiorkor

(big bellies due to liver enlargement)

What physical findings are special tipoffs to protein malnutrition?

- Hepatomegaly

- Dependent edema (low albumin)

- Dry, light-colored, brittle hair

Strict vegetarians (vegan) may need supplementation of which vitamins or minerals?

B12 (most often tested!)
Iron
Calcium & vitamin D
Zinc

How can vegetarians improve their absorption of iron from vegetable sources?

Consume iron with vitamin C (increases transport)

When do infants with malrotation usually present?

First month of life

What is the most common *identifiable* cause of chronic gastritis in kids?

H. pylori

If a child develops nausea, vomiting, and peripheral edema following a viral illness, what should you suspect?

Menetrier disease
(protein-losing gastropathy)

What usually causes Menetrier disease?

CMV

How does the stomach look on endoscopy in Menetrier disease?

Swollen & folded

What is the usual course for Menetrier disease in children?

Spontaneous resolution over months (in adults it is chronic)

How common is it for *normal* infants to pass meconium in the first 24 h of life?

Very **common –**
94 % in first day
98 % in the first 2 days

What GI side effect is vincristine especially known for?	Small bowel ileus
Is rotavirus vaccination routinely recommended for young children in daycare?	Yes – It is generally given at 2, 4, & 6 months (an earlier version of the vaccine increased the incidence of intussusception, the current one does not appear to)
A "sausage-shaped" mass in the right upper abdomen is the buzz phrase for what diagnosis?	**Intussusception** **(the "sausage" is palpable on physical exam and is also sometimes seen via radiology)**
If an intussusception occurs, how long will it take for the bowel to die (usually)?	24 h
In which seasons is intussusception most likely to occur?	Fall & spring
In kids, do you expect pain with a peptic ulcer perforation?	No (for some reason that's really not clear!)
For young children (<2 years old) with vomiting, slow growth, and GI bleeding, but no evidence of abdominal pain, what diagnosis should you suspect?	Peptic ulcer disease
What is odynophagia?	Pain with swallowing
How is an anal fissure treated?	**Good hygiene** **&** **Sitz baths**
Where are anal fissures nearly always found?	**In the midline (90 %)**
How do anal fissures present?	**Rectal bleeding** **&** **Sharp pain with bowel movements**

What does "asterixis" on physical exam suggest?	Hepatic encephalopathy
What is asterixis?	Involuntary "flapping," if the patient holds his or her wrist up in dorsiflexion
What causes hepatic encephalopathy?	**High ammonia levels (due to liver dysfunction)**
What other problem is sometimes mistaken for hepatic encephalopathy and is more likely to be a problem for patients with poor liver function?	**Hypoglycemia**
What stressors are likely to throw a liver patient into hepatic encephalopathy? (5 items – acronym spells LIVER)	Librium or other sedatives Infection Volume loss Electrolyte disturbance *RBC load in the gut (especially common)*
How is hepatic encephalopathy treated? (3 items)	1. Decrease protein in diet/control GI bleeding 2. Give lactulose 3. Oral or rectal neomycin
What metabolic condition makes the symptoms of hepatic encephalopathy worse?	Alkalosis
How can processes within the liver cause elevated conjugated bilirubin?	• Damage to liver cells (that still allows bile to be conjugated) • Damage to biliary endothelium
Which type of bilirubin turns the urine dark – excess conjugated or excess unconjugated bilirubin?	Conjugated

Chapter 4
General Vitamin and Nutrition Question and Answer Items

What is the most reliable way to determine whether a child is getting adequate calories and nutrition?	3–5 days of *prospective* diet history
What "special conditions" must be fulfilled to make a prospective diet history valid?	**Must include at least 1 weekend day** **Must be completed when the child is well**
Which aspects of the physical exam are especially important, when nutritional issues are suspected? (5)	1. Hair 2. Skin 3. Oral mucosa 4. SubQ fat 5. Muscle mass
How is measuring height & weight a little like checking BP for hypertension?	*Three measurements* are required (use the average)
Until what age should you definitely use length, rather than height?	2 years
Is the expected growth pattern different for breastfed vs. formula-fed infants?	• Yes
If so, do you expect differences in length, weight, or both?	• Both

C.M. Houser, *Pediatric Gastroenterology and Nutrition: A Practically Painless Review*, 133
DOI 10.1007/978-1-4939-0449-5_4, © Springer Science+Business Media New York 2014

If a child is described as "wasted" (and he or she hasn't been doing drugs or alcohol!), what does that mean?

The child is skinny – underweight for height

(think of the appearance in adult AIDS patients – it was originally called the "wasting disease" in Africa)

If a child is described as "stunted," what does that mean?

The child is short due to nutritional issues –

The proportions are normal, however. Not particularly "skinny" for their height

What are the most sensitive growth parameters you can use when evaluating for malnutrition?
(2)

Weight *gain* & growth *velocity*

Malnutrition in an otherwise healthy kid with good access to food could be important because _____?

May be the presenting sign of a chronic disease
(IBD, malignancy, etc.)

How is body mass index (BMI) calculated?

Weight/height^2

(kg/m^2)

Why is BMI a useful tool in nutritional research?

The BMI number has good correlation with a person's mass (how big they are) but not much correlation with height – so it's a good measure of how large the person is

(not used in infants)

At what BMI should you consider a child to be overweight?

85–94 % for age & sex

(*Note that the "overweight" category can also include children with high lean body mass and therefore higher weight than usual for height – it is not a measure of adiposity*)

At what BMI is a child considered obese?

≥ 95 % for age & sex

Is zinc absorbed as easily from formulas as it is from human milk?	Generally, no
How do formula-fed babies get sufficient zinc?	The amount of zinc in the formula is increased to compensate for decreased absorption (usually)
Zinc is only about 25 % available in soy formulas – why so low?	"Phytates" inhibit zinc absorption (phytates are a component of soy)
Do infants fed soy-based formulas have lower zinc levels than infants fed cow milk-based formulas?	Yes
Do premature infants have different zinc needs compared to term infants?	Yes – higher
Phytates are thought to decrease absorption of which minerals?	Zinc Iron Calcium Phosphorus (remember that phytates are found in soy preparations)
Are nutritional requirements for commercial formulas voluntary in the USA or required by law?	Required by law – Infant Formula Act of 1980
What is the ratio of calcium:phosphorus supposed to be in commercial formulas?	1:5
If preterm infants have a higher than typical need for zinc, is their need for calcium and phosphorus also high?	Yes
If a preterm infant is exclusively breastfed, will he or she need mineral supplements?	Yes – Zinc, calcium, and phos
What is the minimum amount of iron in commercial formulas?	1 mg iron/L
How much iron is typically available in breast milk?	0.3 mg iron/L

If a formula is designated "iron forti-fied," how much iron will it contain?	10–12 mg iron/L
How do exclusively breastfed infants get enough iron, if the amount in breast milk is so low? (2)	1. The bioavailability is higher 2. Fetal/neonatal iron stores last for 4–6 months
What is "rachitic rosary?"	A series of round, enlarged areas where the ribs meet the sternum – looks a little like a string of rosary beads
What disorder does your patient probably have if you see a rachitic rosary?	Rickets (Vitamin D deficiency due to any cause)
How are chronic hepatitis and a "rachitic rosary" related?	Liver dysfunction can → vitamin D deficiency & rickets
Which medication increases both metabolism & excretion of vitamin D?	Phenobarbital (also stimulates biliary flow)
How would biliary obstruction affect vitamin D absorption?	It impairs absorption (bile salts & micelles needed to solubilize it)
Which class of medications can interfere with vitamin D absorption (& absorption of other fat-soluble vitamins, too) – based on its intraluminal action?	Bile acid binders (e.g., cholestyramine)
Why might chronic liver disease lead to osteoporosis?	Vitamin D malabsorption/inadequate processing
How common is osteoporosis in children with chronic liver disease?	Common – About 2/3
If chronic liver disease is causing rickets or osteoporosis, how can this be treated?	Give 25-hydroxy-vitamin D (oral or parenteral, depending on the problem)
Why might cystic fibrosis patients have back pain and poor posture?	**Vertebral wedge fractures due to osteoporosis (secondary to poor vit D absorption)**

If a cystic fibrosis patient loses his or her deep tendon reflexes and has difficulty with coordination, ptosis, and ophthalmoplegia, what would you guess is the problem?

Vitamin E deficiency

Oculobulbar muscle dysfunction, loss of vibration & position sense, muscle weakness, and truncal ataxia go with which nutritional problem?

Vitamin E deficiency

Are the problems of vitamin E deficiency reversible, when adequate amounts of vitamin E are given?

Yes, *if corrected before age 5 years*

Which types of nutritional molecules are most often deficient among CF patients?

(3 groups)

Fat-soluble vitamins
Metal ions
Essential fatty acids

When vitamin D deficiency develops in CF patients, do those patients usually present in early childhood or later?

Typically in adolescence or later

What are the two main reasons CF patients don't absorb fat and fat-related molecules very well?

(2 reasons)

• Exocrine pancreatic dysfunction

• Increased fecal loss of bile acids

What rather general group of signs indicates essential fatty acid deficiency?
(4 groups)

Skin desquamation
Poor wound healing
Growth failure
Poor immune function/frequent infections

Muscle cramping and weakness + hyperreflexia, & Trousseau's sign = what deficiency?

(Trousseau's sign is carpopedal spasm when you inflate the BP cuff, cutting off arterial flow)

Magnesium

(Calcium deficiency/hypocalcemia is usually associated with Trousseau's sign; it is seen in low magnesium because magnesium is a cofactor for calcium metabolism)

Are CF patients at risk for magnesium deficiency?

Yes –
Due to malabsorption and other factors

Purpuric skin lesions and unexpected GI bleeding suggest what deficiency?	**Vitamin K**
Dry skin, trouble seeing at night, anemia, and dry eyes suggest what deficiency?	**Vitamin A**
What is a Bitot spot?	**A collection of keratin in the bulbar conjunctiva (vitamin A deficiency)**
What does a Bitot spot look like?	A dry silver-gray spot on the conjunctiva
What are the three main body systems for which vitamin A is critical?	**Eye/vision** **Skin/epithelial surfaces** **Immune system**
What are the two main functions of vitamin A for the eyes?	1. **Critical part of the light perception molecule** 2. **Maintains healthy epithelia for the conjunctiva & cornea**
If sufficient vitamin A is not available, what happens to the body's epithelial tissues?	**They dry, and mucus-related epithelia turns into squamous & keratinized epithelia**
	Mnemonic: Think of the side effects of isotretinoin to help you remember this!
If a child is vitamin A deficient and contracts a routine illness such as pneumonia, diarrhea, or measles, how much more likely is that child to die compared to a child with adequate vitamin A?	**25 %**

How is vitamin A deficiency evaluated in terms of labs?
                (2 options)
	Plasma retinol level
	                OR
	Retinol-binding protein (RBP)
	(cheaper option)

Vitamin A is famous for being found in carrots. Where else is dietary vitamin A found?

(2 sources)

1. Any dark orange fruit
2. Dark green leafy veggies

What purpose does copper have in hematology?

It is needed to produce normal hemoglobin

(*converts ferrous iron to ferric iron*)

What effect does copper deficiency have on the CBC?

Microcytic, hypochromic anemia

Which kids are especially likely to become copper deficient based on their diet?

TPN kids – especially if the child has liver disease
(the copper content is often lowered for liver disease, but sometimes it's too much)
&
Infants fed unmodified cow's milk

What is the most appropriate use of the BMI?

**Obesity screening –
it is both valid & reliable for this purpose**

What are the four sites typically used to measure skin folds?

1. **Bicep**
2. **Tricep**
3. **Subscapular
(think of it as the bra line fat roll)**
4. **Suprailiac
(the "love handle" fat roll)**

How consistent are skin fold measurements made at different times or by different people?

Not consistent

How good is the correlation between total body fat and skin fold measurements?

Not good

What important body fat store do skin fold measurements completely miss?

Intraabdominal fat

At what age should children's height be measured standing rather than lying down?	**>2 years old**
What is the name of the device used to most accurately obtain height measurements?	**A stadiometer** **(still need three measurements, though)**
What is the least expensive and most useful lab test for evaluating nutritional status?	CBC
What is primary malnutrition?	Inadequate calorie intake
What is secondary malnutrition?	Calorie intake would normally be adequate, but something else is getting in the way (malabsorption, nutrient losses, abnormally high need for nutrients)
What does "protein–energy malnutrition" refer to?	Deficit of protein *or* overall calories – either one (there is significant overlap in the disorders, so they are sometimes referred to jointly this way)
Protein malnutrition (alone) is called _____?	Kwashiorkor
Inadequate calorie malnutrition is called _____?	Marasmus
Is it possible to have both marasmus and kwashiorkor?	Of course – calorie deficit & inadequate protein "marasmic kwashiorkor"
Is malnutrition known to cause selective deficits in immune cell populations?	**Yes – T cells are selectively decreased in protein–energy malnutrition**
If you note lymphopenia in a malnourished patient, what should you assume is the likely source of the lymphopenia?	Low T cell count

How do you calculate the total lymphocyte count?

WBC count

×

% lymphocytes in CBC

If your patient has moderate-to-severe protein–energy malnutrition, and you place a PPD, what problem might you have in interpreting the results?

These patients are often _anergic_ due to low T cell counts

(any delayed-type hypersensitivity reaction will be affected)

Which commonly measured plasma proteins are acute-phase reactants?

Albumin & prealbumin

In the presence of a catabolic stressor, what happens to the albumin or the prealbumin level?

It goes **down**

(Positive acute-phase reactants go up with catabolic stresses, e.g., CRP. Negative acute-phase reactants go down with catabolic stress)

Which body protein is the cheapest and easiest one to measure?

Albumin

What aspects of albumin make it less than ideal as a way to measure a patient's protein status?
(3)

- **Long half-life (20 days)**
- **>50 % of albumin is normally extravascular – when serum levels decline, albumin from other parts of the body will boost the level to make protein balance seem normal**
- **It's an acute-phase reactant**

What factors, other than protein supply, affect the level of visceral protein found in the blood?
(4)

(visceral proteins = proteins synthesized by body organs, like albumin)

1. **Synthesis problems (e.g., liver disease or aging)**
2. **Increased losses (e.g., burns, protein-losing enteropathy)**
3. **Fluid overload**
4. **Redistribution to other body spaces (e.g., capillary leak syndromes)**

How is prealbumin related to albumin?

It is similar in size and charge – otherwise not related

(In other words, they end up close together on an electrophoresis gel)

What kind of molecule is prealbumin?	A transport molecule for thyroxine (its other name is "transthyretin")
What is the best serum marker of nutritional status?	**Prealbumin**
Why is prealbumin a better measure of nutrition status than albumin? (2 reasons)	• **Short half-life of 2 days** • **Requires significant supply of essential amino acids to make it** **(these factors make prealbumin level more responsive to changes in nutrition)**
Which patients in clinical practice are likely to be hypermetabolic?	Hospitalized & acutely ill patients (chronically ill may also have elevated metabolism)
Which large pediatric patient group is often hypometabolic?	Mentally retarded
What is a "conditionally essential" nutrient? (should really be called an "optimizing" nutrient)	A nutrient that is not essential for a particular body function but nonetheless *improves clinical or metabolic outcomes when supplements are given*
What are some classic examples of conditionally essential nutrients? (3 examples)	Folate (neural tube defects) Vitamin A (↓ mortality from infectious disease) Zinc (↓ diarrheal & respiratory infections)
What is a "neutraceutical?"	A nutrient or other biological material used in high/pharmacological doses (example is giving lactobacilli)
There are several different types of nutrition recommendations. As a group, they can all be referred to as _____?	Dietary Reference Intakes (DRIs)
What is the "most appropriate measure" to use when evaluating a patient's nutrient intake?	**The Recommended Daily Allowance (RDA)**

What is an RDA?	The daily amount of a nutrient needed to *prevent deficiency* in 98 % of the population
If a patient's diet does not meet the RDA for a particular nutrient, can you conclude that the patient is deficient for that nutrient?	No – individual's needs vary
What is a UI?	Tolerable upper intake level – the largest amount of a nutrient that is not likely to cause a health problem for most people
	(created due to all those health food retailers selling megadoses of vitamins!!)
What are RDIs and DRVs in general terms? (Reference Daily Intake & Daily Reference Values)	The food values on food packaging – intended for consumer use
The nutritional figures on food packaging are based on a daily diet of how many calories?	2,000–2,500
Breastfed babies with strict vegetarian mothers are at risk for what dietary deficiency?	**B12**
At what age can infants be fed regular cow's milk?	12 months – (cow's milk is a frequent cause of occult GI bleeding before 12 months)
What vitamin supplement is recommended for all breastfed infants?	**Vitamin D**
What are the guidelines for when vitamin D supplementation should be given to breastfed infants?	Preterm infants: 2 months of age Full term: 4–6 months old
Why do most breastfeeding mothers who stop breast-feeding in the first few weeks make that choice?	"Lack of support" for breastfeeding and dealing with common lactation problems

In the first few weeks after a mother's milk has come in, is it alright to supplement feedings with bottle feedings?	**No – It disrupts the feeding routine and will decrease successful breastfeeding**
If infants seem "colicky" or parents complain of vague GI problems in their infant, should formulas be switched to improve the symptoms?	**No**
If a mother elects <u>not</u> to breast-feed, how should you, as a pediatrician or other healthcare professional, respond?	Supportive & nonjudgemental (assuming that she had the benefit of positive information about breastfeeding)
Which hormone is responsible for milk letdown?	Oxytocin (stimulated by infant sucking on nipple, infant's cry, etc.)
Which hormone is responsible for milk production?	<u>PRO</u>lactin (like <u>PRO</u>duction)
Common causes of decreased milk production are _____? (3 causes)	1. Maternal fatigue 2. Stress 3. Certain medications
Common causes of decreased milk-ejection reflex/letdown are _____?	1. Pain 2. Distraction 3. Fatigue
If a baby does not feed well, or regularly, in the first few days of life, what is the impact on breastfeeding success?	Usually none
Regular feeding routines are most important after what maternal physiological event?	**Initial change from colostrum to milk**
How often will most newborn babies feed?	Every 2–3 h
How long is <u>too</u> long for a newborn to go between feedings?	**5 h (even 4 h is a long time)**

Which group of infants feeds more often, breast fed or bottle fed?	Breast fed (Breast milk is processed more rapidly)
Current recommendations suggest what pattern of breastfeeding in the first postpartum days?	10–15-min feeding on <u>each</u> breast at <u>each</u> feeding
Are the motor skills needed for breastfeeding and bottle feeding quite similar or quite different?	Quite different
Although a regular feeding schedule is important for both the infant's needs and successful breastfeeding, do current guidelines recommend following a set schedule (based on the clock)?	No – "regular" but "not rigid" are the buzzwords
If a breastfeeding mother complains of discomfort during feedings, and would like to shorten feeds, how should you respond?	Decreasing the amount the baby eats will lead to milk involution and possibly inadequate infant nutrition
Are creams & ointments helpful for nipple pain with breastfeeding?	No (Sources vary about this)
If the breasts are engorged with milk, what will improve the discomfort?	Expression of milk (According to pediatric materials, a hand pump can be used. Most obs recommend strongly against these due to nipple pain/damage with their use)
Nipple pain with breastfeeding is most often due to what three problems?	1. Incorrect positioning of infant 2. Forgetting to break suction before removing the critter 3. Too little areola in the mouth
If Mom notices that the interval between feedings is shrinking, should she be worried that junior isn't getting enough to eat?	No – it usually signifies a growth spurt (more frequent feeds allow the baby to get more food & boost milk production, too)
Infants commonly lose how much of their birth weight in the first few days of life?	10 % (regained by 2 weeks, generally)

Most infant formulas are mainly composed of _____?	Skim milk
What is the carbohydrate source in most infant formula?	**Lactose**
What is the carbohydrate source in premature infant formulas?	**Corn syrup solids**
What is the fat source in infant formulas?	**Vegetable oils**
What are the negative aspects of soy-based formulas? (3 aspects)	1. High aluminum levels 2. LBW infants/preemies don't tolerate well 3. Infants with allergies to cow's milk often have allergic reactions to soy, also
What group of infants will most clearly benefit from soy products?	**Those with transient lactase deficiency after a diarrheal illness**
Is the nutritional content of soy-based and milk-based formulas equivalent?	Yes
What is the carbohydrate source in soy-based formulas?	**Sucrose/corn syrup**
Should bottles used by infants be sterilized?	No – Soap & water washing is fine (dishwasher is even better)
When do infants usually wean from bottle to cup?	By about 1 year
How much is the average newborn expected to eat?	**2–3 oz every 2–3 h**
After the first week of life, how much will the average infant usually eat?	2–4 oz every 2–4 h
Must formula be sterilized by the parents before feeding it to a newborn?	No

Formula should not make up more than __% of an infant's total calories at 6 months?	65 % (<30 oz)
Is it alright to give infants a bottle just before bedtime?	**Yes**
Is it alright to give infants a bottle to take into the crib with them at bedtime?	**No –** **Big risk of dental caries**
If an infant is breast fed, but also takes supplemental formula feedings, should he or she still receive vitamin D supplements?	**Depends –** **<500 ccs of formula per day still needs vit D supplements**
How much vitamin D supplement should you give to infants?	**400 IU/day**
Why is vitamin D now recommended for all exclusively breast-fed infants?	**Increased risk of rickets was noted** **(even with supposedly good sunlight exposure)**
Should children and adolescents take vitamin D supplements?	Yes, _if_ 1. Inadequate sunlight exposure 2. Don't take an MVI with 600 IU/day 3. Don't drink ≥750 ccs fortified milk per day
In addition to vitamin D supplementation, exclusively breast-fed full-term infants also need supplementation of what other vitamin/mineral as they get older?	**Iron at 4–6 months**
At what age will the premature infant require iron supplementation?	1 month old
How should iron supplementation be dosed for full-term infants?	**1 mg/kg/day elemental iron**
How can iron supplements be provided to infants? (3 ways)	1. Fortified formula 2. Fortified cereal 3. Ferrous sulfate drops

If fluoride supplementation is needed, at what age should it be started?

6 months
(or a bit older)
Depending on water concentration of fluoride

What level of fluoride in the water supply means that supplementation is not needed?

>0.6 Parts per million (PPM)

Is too much fluoride a problem?

Yes, but quite rare –
It causes "fluorosis"

What is "fluorosis?"

"Mottled enamel" on the teeth
&
Osteosclerosis of the bones

(fluoride replaces calcium in these tissues)

In what circumstance should you wait to supplement fluoride until the child is 3 years old?

Medium concentration of fluoride in the water
(0.3–0.6 PPM)

Are the rules for fluoride supplementation different for breast-fed vs. bottle-fed kids?

No

(Fluoride the Mom drinks will be in the breast milk)

When should solid foods be started?

4–6 months

Which solid foods are usually added first?

Cereals

Which foods are usually added to the diet last?

Meats

What three types of items are often held until after 12 months due to the potential for allergic responses in younger children?
           (4 types)

1. Eggs
2. Fish/seafood
3. Wheat
4. Nuts

Cow's milk may be added after what age?

12 months

What type of cow's milk should be given to infants and why?	• **Whole milk** • **The fat & cholesterol requirement for development in this period is high**
By what age should children be switched to skim or 2 % milk?	**2 years**
What is the recommended pattern for introduction of <u>each</u> new food item?	**Give a single new item, wait for 3–5 days before introducing another**
For the first 2 years of life, fat should make up what percentage of the total calories?	**About 40 %**
Infants & young toddlers should avoid what unfortunately shaped foods?	**Things shaped like the airway – especially if they're firm (For example, grapes, peanuts, hard candy)**
Is it alright to give infants/toddlers popcorn if they are old enough to be eating corn products?	**No – still an aspiration risk**
What's wrong with feeding toddlers hotdogs?	<u>**Whole**</u> **or** <u>**sliced**</u> **hotdogs can occlude the airway**
Raw fruit and vegetables are good for people, in general. Are they good for toddlers?	**Yes, if they are cut up – large pieces are an aspiration risk**
Assuming that <u>you</u> don't have to eat with the child, should you encourage self-feeding?	Yes
According to the ABP, is it a good idea for very young children to snack between meals?	No – "grazing" is discouraged
What are the "ingredients" of a good toddler meal according to the ABP?	1. Family sits together 2. No TV 3. Self-feeding 4. Set duration (such as 30 min)

If an infant is constipated, is iron-fortified formula a likely culprit?	**No (especially not on board questions!)**
The most common deficiency of essential fatty acids is _____?	**Linoleic acid**
Essential fatty acid deficiency causes what sort of symptoms & signs?	**Diarrhea** **Dermatitis** **Hair loss** **(typical signs of nutrition problems)**
Infants with congenital heart disease are at risk for what nutritional issue (the main issue, that is)?	Inadequate calories (because they are fluid restricted & have high calorie needs)
How do you calculate calorie needs, per day, based on weight?	**100/kg – First 10 kg** **50/kg – Second 10 kg** **20/kg – any additional kgs** **(Similar to calculating fluid needs!)**
How much iron is in regular commercial formulas?	**12 mg/L**
Do artificial flavors & colors contribute to the development of ADHD?	No documented role
What is the most common cause of urticaria & angioedema in kids?	**Artificial flavors & colors**
What are the two most <u>common</u> complications of NG feeding?	1. **Diarrhea (most common)** 2. **GE reflux (second most common)**
Is the diarrhea associated with NG feeding likely to lead to dehydration?	**No (it's generally not severe)**
The most <u>severe</u> or <u>worst</u> complication of NG feedings in infants is _____?	**Aspiration or vomiting with aspiration**
How can you reduce the risk of diarrhea & reflux with NG feeds in terms of the type of formula you give?	Give elemental formula

Ostomy feedings have what additional complication possibility, which NG feedings do not have? (Ostomy Refeeding?)

Infection of the wou.

A common cause of iron deficiency anemia in toddlers/older infants is _____?

Too much cow's milk

If an infant has an allergy to milk, what type of formula should you switch to?

Elemental

(there is a lot of cross-reactivity with soy, so it is *not* a good choice)

NG feeds can be given as a bolus or continuously. Which is better for congenital heart disease babies, and why?

**Continuous –
High calorie need combined with slow gastric emptying & rapid satiety makes continuous better**

What is the main nutritional goal for an infant with congenital heart disease prior to correction?

Fatten 'em up – Get them ready for surgery ASAP
(gain as much weight as possible)

In addition to infants with congenital heart disease, which other infants will benefit from continuous feeds?
(3)

1. **Reflux kids**
2. **Crohn's disease**
3. **Malabsorption syndromes**

Which vitamin deficiencies are most common in preemies?

**Fat solubles (ADEK) –
Because they don't produce much bile acid**

In addition to fat-soluble vitamins, what other dietary fat is difficult to absorb if you don't make much bile acid?

Long-chain triglycerides

(so preemies have trouble getting enough of these, also)

What is the most common cause of obesity?

Overeating

What are clues to whether a child's obesity is due to overeating vs. hormones/genetics?

Overeating → tall height & advanced bone age

Hormonal/genetic causes → short height & delayed bone age

boards vignette indicates that a ...ld is obese, but the vital informa-...on about bone age isn't given, you ...ould consider what possible endocrine cause?	**Cushing's syndrome**
What are the three most likely endocrine causes of obesity?	1. **Hypothyroidism** 2. **Cushing's** 3. **Growth hormone deficiency**
What is the most typical genetic cause of obesity?	**Prader–Willi**
What is the definition of overweight?	BMI 85th–94th percentile for age & gender (>85 % is "at risk" for obesity) Overweight: 85th–94th percentile Obese: ≥95th percentile
What is the definition of obesity in a child?	BMI ≥ 95th percentile for age & gender
A <u>tall</u> obese child is probably obese due to _____?	**Overeating** **(sometimes called "exogenous obesity")**
If a child is obese at age 6 years, how likely is he or she to be obese as an adult?	**25 %**
If a child is obese at age 12 years, what is the likelihood that he or she will be obese as an adult?	**75 %**
An obese child with advanced bone age is probably obese due to _____?	**Overeating** **(exogenous obesity)**
Is genetics important in the development of obesity?	**Yes**
In terms of fat distribution, how important is genetics in determining the distribution?	Very – about 75 % of the variation in fat distribution is due to genetics

What is the strongest evidence for genetics' role in adult weight?

Identical twins reared apart <u>still</u> end up with similar weights as adults

A short child with delayed bone age and obesity should be evaluated for which causes of obesity?

Genetic & hormonal

The best way, generally speaking, to reduce adult obesity is to do what in pediatrics?

Prevent childhood obesity

What is the only effective weight loss program for children? (Success rate is still not great)

Diet
Exercise
Behavior modification

Should fenfluramine or dextrofenfluramine be prescribed for children having difficulty losing weight?

No!

(Not used in adults anymore, either!)

How does sibutramine (Meridia™) work to reduce weight?

Slight increase in temperature burns calories

What are the typical side effects for sibutramine (Meridia™)?

Tachycardia & HTN *(Drug withdrawn from US market due to cardiovascular risks).*

How does orlistat (Xenical™) reduce weight?

Blocks fat absorption

What is the main side effect of orlistat?

Diarrhea with fatty meals!

How is "weight maintenance" used to manage obesity in children?

If an obese child has not yet had its growth spurt, maintaining the current weight through the growth spurt will often correct the problem

Some popular press articles argue that obesity does not cause significant health risks. Are there significant health risks documented with obesity?

Yes

What psychiatric disorder is associated with obesity?

Depression

What cardiovascular conditions are clearly associated with obesity?

Hypertension
&
Coronary artery disease

Which orthopedic disorders are clearly linked to obesity?
(One adult & three childhood disorders)

1. **Osteoarthritis**
2. **Avascular necrosis of the femoral head**
3. **SCFE**
4. **Blount's disease**
(tibial bowing & abnormalities)

Obesity is clearly linked to what two common pulmonary disorders?

1. **Asthma (increased inflammatory mediators)**
2. **Sleep apnea**

(also contributes to pulmonary hypertension)

Among endocrine disorders, DM type 2 and polycystic ovarian syndrome are clearly related to what weight issue?

Obesity!

If a vignette presents a female adolescent with unusually high or low weight for initial evaluation, what "touchy-feely" answer is often the board looking for?

"Ask her how she thinks about her weight"

If one parent is obese, what is the probability that any children of the pair will also be obese?

50 %
(roughly – sources vary)

If both parents are obese, what is the probability that their children will be obese?

75 %
(roughly – sources vary)

Breast-fed premature infants often require supplementation of what basic dietary component?

Protein

Preterm infants receive a smaller amount of milk from their breastfeeding mothers in the first month. How does the composition of the milk help to make up for this?

It has a higher concentration of fat, protein, vitamins A & E, and NaCl

How long after the birth
of a preterm infant will the mother's
milk approximate a full-term
mother's milk?

At about 1 month postpartum

**Full-term infants require how much
protein per day, in the first 6 months,
for good growth and development?**

2.5 g/kg/day

**Preemies have an increased need
for protein, until they have made
up the growth they expected to do
in utero. How much is their protein
requirement?**

3.5 g/kg/day

Why is colostrum yellow?

Large amounts of carotene

Is colostrum beneficial for the gut?

Yes – two reasons:
1. **Stimulates it to pass meconium**
2. **Stimulates gut maturation/
   processing of fats**

**Colostrum is especially high in what
dietary component?**

Protein

**One part of the protein found in
colostrum is _____ from the
immune system?**

Immunoglobulins

(mainly IgA)

**Board exams are very big on your
knowing that the "hind" (or last part
of the milk) is higher in what dietary
component than the early milk
("foremilk")?**

Fat (& also protein)

Mnemonic: <u>H</u>ind is <u>H</u>igher in fat

**Human breast milk is low in what
important vitamin?**

**Vitamin K
(contributes to neonatal/newborn
hemorrhage issues)**

**Why do neonates have trouble with
low levels of vitamin K?**
                (2 reasons)

1. **Doesn't cross placenta well**
2. **Made in the gut by bacteria –
   newborns don't have a well-
   developed collection of bacteria
   in their gut yet!**

Human breast milk is quite low in what dietary component?

**Protein –
1/3 the amount in cow's milk**

Why is IgA from colostrum or breast milk important?

It provides "local immunity" – this means that it binds toxins/bacteria present in the food or the gut

What is the protein content of cow's milk?

**3 %
(Not as high as you might think!)**

What is the protein content of human milk?

**1 %

(Remember, it's 1/3 of cow's milk)**

The sugar source in breast milk is which sugar?

Lactose

What is the main calorie source in commercially prepared formulas?

Lactose

(Breast milk & commercial formulas have the same calorie source)

What is the calorie content of breast milk or commercial formulas?
(They are the same)

20 kcal/oz

(same as 2/3 kcal per cc)

What is the fat content of cow's milk?

Also about 3 % –
Like protein content

What is the fat content of mother's milk?

Varies with diet, but similar to cow's milk

How are the casein and whey ratios related in mother's milk vs. cow's milk?

They are the inverse of each other

What is the ratio of casein:whey in mother's milk?

80:20

**Mnemonic:
Only a human could be "casing" a joint, so human milk is mostly casein
Think of an 80-year-old human casing the joint, if you have trouble remembering the 80 %**

If human milk is 80 % casein, what is the casein:whey ratio for cow's milk?

20:80

Which has more iron, breast milk or formula?	**Formula**
Why is the iron content of an infant's food not terribly important in the first 4 months of life?	**Iron stores from the fetal period are sufficient for the first 4 months**
Which one has the best bioavailability of iron – breast milk or formula?	**Breast milk**
If you are asked which one is a <u>better iron source,</u> breast milk or formula, which should you answer?	**Breast milk (due to better absorption)**
Is iron absorbed better from breast milk or from formula?	**Breast milk**
Although the iron in breast milk has better bioavailability than the iron in formula, which has a bigger iron content?	Formula (The net result is that the formula-fed baby gets more iron)
In a vignette, a new mother complains that her newborn isn't growing. The newborn is gaining 20–30 g/day (after losing weight in the first few days of life). What should you do?	**Reassure**
Approximately what is the calorie requirement of a newborn?	**120 kcal/kg/day**
If a board question gives important information in pounds, how do you convert to kilos?	**2.2 lb = 1 kg**
If an infant is not sleeping through the night, will advancing to solids help him/her to sleep longer?	**No**
What is the connection between early introduction of solids and children's weight at older ages?	Linked to obesity (supposedly due to the high calorie content of solid foods)

Why might a young infant
(<6 months old) have difficulty
digesting solid foods?

Low levels of amylase
(amylase is needed to digest starch
properly)

**What is the relationship between
early introduction of solids
and the immune system?**

**Allergies are more likely if solids are
introduced while the immune system
is immature**

20–30 g/day is the expected rate
for weight gain of an infant fitting
what description?

Average full-term newborn
(after the first few days of life,
of course)

**What is the expected weight gain
for a premature infant?**

**15–20 g/day
(based on a 120 kcal/kg/day diet)**

**Which of the two malnutrition
syndromes does the board
usually test?**

**Kwashiorkor
(protein malnutrition – total calories
may be adequate)**

**What are the hallmarks
of kwashiorkor?**

1. **"Pot belly" (significantly distended,
   like on the TV commercials for
   African charities)**
2. **Pitting edema (due to low protein)
   Brittle hair and sometimes rash**

**In what settings does kwashiorkor
most often develop?**

1. **Developing nations**
2. **Refugee camps**
3. **Communes – if it's a vegetarian
   commune (rare in actual practice,
   more common on board exams)**

How can you remember that
kwashiorkor is <u>protein</u> malnutrition?

"Kwash" sounds like "squash" which
has almost no protein

In case you get confused, how can
you remember that marasmus is due
to overall low calories?

If you were stuck in a "morass" (think
of a big swamp with quicksand), you
would be lacking just about everything!

If a child is drinking only vegetable-based
milk sources, what disorder may develop?

Kwashiorkor

**How is the clinical presentation
of marasmus different from
kwashiorkor?**

**No edema
No pot belly
Hair is fairly normal**

(3)

**Marasmus doesn't create most
of the problems of kwashiorkor,
so what happens in this disorder?**

**Underweight children/adults
with muscle wasting**

(both disorders have muscle wasting)

**Rickets can develop when children
have problems in what two organs
(other than the gut or the skin)?**

**Liver
  Or
Kidney**

**On the boards, rickets is sometimes
presented with liver disease. Why
would liver disease cause rickets, in
terms of absorption issues?**

**Inadequate production of bile acids
decreases absorption of the fat-soluble
vitamins
(including vitamin D)**

**Why would renal disease/renal failure
cause rickets?**

**The kidney processes vitamin D into
its active form**

**What are the four forms
of vitamin D?**

D_2 = **ergocalciferol (in milk)**

D_3 = **cholecalciferol (sun-exposed
skin – think of the cholesterol
in the skin cell membranes
to remember "cholecalciferol")**

25-OH D_3 = storage form

1,25 (OH)$_2$ D_3 = active form

Which enzyme is considered to
be the most important part of the
vitamin D regulation system?

1-hydroxylase in the kidney

What determines the activity
of the critical kidney enzyme in the
vitamin D synthesis pathway?
(4 items)

1. Serum calcium
2. Serum phosphate
3. PTH
4. $1\alpha,25(OH)_2D_3$

**What is the main source
of vitamin D for humans?**

Photochemical conversion

**If adequate sunshine is available,
is there *any* dietary requirement
for vitamin D?**

No

Where in the body is vitamin D stored?
(3)

Blood
Adipose tissue
Muscle tissue

Vitamin D protects skin cells from some environmental damage and can also be given as a topical treatment for which disorder?

Psoriasis
(Vitamin D analogs are used)

What little known endocrine effect of vitamin D is related to diabetes?

Induces insulin secretion by pancreas

Are dark-skinned individuals at increased risk of vitamin D deficiency?

Yes –
Especially if they live in colder (darker) environments

If dietary vitamin D is not needed, then how are the vitamin D diet requirements formulated?

They assume very little light exposure (which means that they may overestimate what is needed by most people)

What are the findings typical of rickets on the chest X-ray?

1. **"Rachitic rosary" (little balls of increased calcium at the costochondral junctions)**
2. **Pigeon chest (sternum protrudes too far)**

How are the effects of vitamin D deficiency different in adults or older children as compared to young children?

Causes "osteomalacia" or soft bones

Which vitamin is also a hormone?

Vitamin D

Which vitamin is very close to being a steroid?

Vitamin D
(one ring is broken open – otherwise it would be a steroid)

In addition to bile acid production, why else might liver damage/ dysfunction produce rickets?

The liver processes D_3 to 25-hydroxy D_3

What are vitamin D's two main effects on bone?

1. Activates osteoblasts to synthesize bone
2. Provides adequate calcium level for bone mineralization

What is vitamin D's main effect on the gut?

To permit absorption of calcium

What craniofacial findings are expected in rickets?
(3)

1. **Delayed closure of sutures/ fontanelles in very young children**
2. **Bad tooth enamel**
3. **Skull thickening/frontal bossing**

Widened ends of the bones at the wrists and ankles, plus bowing of the long bones = what disorder?

Rickets

Skull thickening is a paradoxical effect of what vitamin deficiency?

Vitamin D

The main consequence of inadequate vitamin D is that the body cannot maintain its _____?

Calcium level

What is craniotabes?

Weak skull bone in infants – so weak that finger pressure can cause indentation

What nutritional disorder can cause craniotabes?

Rickets

Craniotabes is also seen in what two non-nutritional situations?

1. Prematurity
2. Cleidocranial dysostosis

What CNS effects can occur with rickets?

Seizures & tetany
Drowsiness

(due to low calcium)

In addition to fortified milk products, what is another excellent source of vitamin D?

Fish oil, and oily types of fish

Do you need dietary sources of vitamin D?

Not if there is adequate sunlight exposure

(about 30 min/day – but don't tell the dairy industry!)

Which hormone has an effect opposite PTH's effect on calcium?

Calcitonin
(from the thyroid)

What is the fancy name for vitamin D2?   Ergocalciferol

(2 c's = D2)

What is the fancy name for vitamin D3?   Cholecalciferol

(3 c's = D3)
(the skin one)

Calcitriol refers to both the active &   Vitamin D
inactive forms of what vitamin?   (25-OH and 1,25-OH versions)

Which vitamin is converted to a   Vitamin D → calcitriol
hormone by the body?

Generally speaking, what   **To elevate serum calcium**
is calcitriol's goal for the body?   **(Gets it out of the bones,**
                                         in through the gut, and
                                         prevents renal excretion)

If you are treating vitamin D   **Both vitamin D & calcium**
deficiency with oral supplements,
what supplements should you give?

How can you assess whether   1. Plasma 25-(OH) cholecalciferol level
a patient's vitamin D level is adequate? 2. Alk phos
    (4: 1 direct & 3 indirect)   3. Bone densitometry
                                         4. Serum calcium level

What are the long-bone hallmarks   **Widened or cupped metaphyses**
of rickets on X-ray?
                                         &

                                         Osteopenia

                                         (bowed long bones, also)

Do patients with rickets have trouble   Yes – they are osteopenic
with frequent fractures?

Rachitic rosary has been mentioned   **Rib flaring**
as possible rib finding in rickets.
What is the other description of a
rickets-related rib abnormality?

What is PTH's effect on serum   It raises it
calcium level?

In vitamin D deficiency, calcium levels are low. Should phosphorus levels be high, low, or normal?	**Also low (unusual – in most conditions PO$_4$ goes up when calcium goes down, and vice versa)**
What lab abnormalities, in addition to low calcium and phosphorus levels, help you to confirm a rickets diagnosis?	1. **↑ Alk phos** 2. **↑ PTH** 3. **↓ Calcitriol** **(aka 25-OH vitamin D)**
Do vitamin D deficiency patients typically have any subjective complaints?	Musculoskeletal pain
What are some good dietary sources of vitamin K?	Milk, live yogurt, egg yolk, dark green leafy vegetables
If a patient is vitamin K deficient, how is vitamin K usually given?	IM
If a neonate is bleeding, and you suspect vitamin K deficiency, how will you treat the infant?	1. **FFP – to fix the clotting factors/ bleeding *now*!** 2. **Vitamin K – to help the liver synthesize the factors needed**
What is the gigantically long formal name for vitamin K?	**Phylloquinone** Mnemonic: Misspell it as Phyllo<u>Kw</u>inone, to remember it is vitamin K
In terms of coag studies, what do you expect to see with vitamin K deficiency?	• **Normal bleeding time (platelets are fine)** • **High PT & PTT (both intrinsic & extrinsic system affected)**
Name two common reasons for vitamin K deficiency in children and adults?	1. Fat malabsorption 2. Broad-spectrum antibiotic use – can kill the gut flora that synthesize vitamin K

Is the vitamin K synthesized
by bacteria in the gut sufficient
for all of a person's vitamin K needs?

No –
Dietary deficiency still leads
to deficiency

(It's not really clear how important
the bacterially synthesized K is –
and it is a different form from the
dietary form, also)

Too much vitamin D can cause what
unusual problem?

Ca/Phos levels too high – precipitates
form, mainly in soft tissues (& sometimes in basal ganglia)

If a patient has too much vitamin D,
will he or she have the usual signs
of hypercalcemia?

Yes

**What are the typical signs
of hypercalcemia?**

**Stones, bones, abdominal moans,
& psychic groans**

1. **kidney stones**
2. **bone pain**
3. **abdominal pain & anorexia**
4. **cognitive or psychiatric changes**

Can vitamin D intoxication &
hypercalcemia come from eating too
much calcium and vitamin D?

Yes, but rare –
Milk-alkali syndrome

How is vitamin D toxicity treated?

Mainly treat the hypercalcemia

(hydration, furosemide, fix any associated electrolyte problems)

Bisphosphonates (the "-dronate" drugs)
may be given to speed recovery & drop
calcium levels faster

Why does too much vitamin D cause
high calcium levels?

High levels activate osteoclasts to resorb
bone & dump calcium into the system

(The bisphosphonate drugs inhibit this
osteoclast activity)

**Beans are a good source
for what two important nutrients?**

Iron & folate

Mnemonic:
I̲F̲ you eat beans, you will get
I̲ron & F̲olate

Yummy foods like dark chocolate,
cocoa, nuts, & molasses are high
in what mineral?

Iron

**Children who are iron deficient
are at a greater risk for what
environmental toxicity?**

**Lead – lack of iron increases gut
absorption of lead**

Iron-deficiency anemia causes a lot
of effects due to the resulting anemia.
What two unexpected consequences
can it have?
(Sensory & musculoskeletal)

Sensory – deafness

Musculoskeletal – Decreased bone
density

**If a child's iron intake has been
adequate, but then rapidly becomes
inadequate, what are the two most
likely underlying causes?**

1. **Rapid growth has increased the
   amount needed**
2. **RBCs are being lost somewhere**

Green tea is a dietary source of what
nutrient, in particular?

Vitamin K

**Which clotting factors are vitamin K
dependent?**

**2, 7, 9, & 10
+ C & S**

Folate deficiency is famous for causing
megaloblastic anemia. What other
problems occur with this deficiency?
(2)

Immunity – decreased cellular immunity

*Psychiatric effects – paranoid &
irritable*

What f̲ruity sources of f̲olate are
available in most diets?

Avocado
Apricots
Melons
Oranges

**Vitamin E deficiency is well known
for causing hemolytic anemia in
premature infants. What sort of
problems does it typically cause
for older children & adults?**

**Hyporeflexia & various other
neurological abnormalities**

What is the main overall biochemical function of vitamin E in the body?

Prevention of "lipid peroxidation" by free radicals
(*antioxidant*)

What are good dietary sources of vitamin E?

Health foodstuff –
Wheat germ
Soybeans
Whole wheat
Nuts, seeds, & DGLVs
(dark green leafy veggies)

What does vitamin E deficiency do to RBCs, and why?

- **Increases RBC fragility**
- **Increases risk of RBC hemolysis because its antioxidant properties are missing**

What is the other name for vitamin E?

Tocopherol

Mnemonic: Mispronounce it as "tocopheerol," to remember it is vitamin E!

Is there more than one type of vitamin E?

Yes –
But only one type is active α-tocopherol

Adequate amounts of which trace element protect against the more severe effects of vitamin E deficiency?

Selenium

If you need to evaluate for vitamin E deficiency based on lab tests, what test should you request?

Plasma tocopherol
(adjusted for blood lipid level)

Adequate amounts of which other vitamin reduces the amount of vitamin E needed by the body?

Vitamin C
(it helps to "regenerate" partially used vitamin E)

Night blindness & dry skin suggest which vitamin deficiency?

**Vitamin A
(aka retinol)**

Deficiency of which vitamin causes pellagra?

**Vitamin B3
(Niacin)**

What are the signs of pellagra?

Diarrhea
Dermatitis
Dementia
& Beefy red glossitis
(tongue inflammation)

Mnemonic:
Think of three D's branded onto a
tongue – which is understandably
inflamed after being branded!

If you put together all of the
symptoms of vitamin B3 deficiency,
what are they?

Diarrhea, Dermatitis,
Dementia, Glossitis

(For the poetry minded:

Fast bowels yield diarrhea & irritation
dermatitis;
Thoughts slowed by Dementia,
And tongue by Glossitis.
Woe is me when I am low on B3!)

What is the other name
for vitamin B1?

Thiamine
(Think "Th1am1ne" to remember
that it's B1!)

Vitamin B1 deficiency can create
two different types of syndromes.
What are they?

- **Ber1ber1 (beriberi)**

- **Wernicke–Korsakoff**

If a patient presents with oculomotor
and gait problems due to a vitamin
deficiency, which vitamin &
syndrome is it?

- **B1**

- **Wernicke–Korsakoff (can also have**
  autonomic, memory, and confusion
  problems)

Although it takes a while to come back,
what lab test can help you confirm
thiamine deficiency?

Erythrocyte transketolase activity

Deficiency of which other B vitamin
(in addition to B1) can sometimes
lead to gait problems?

- **B12**

What differentiates the lower extremity symptoms of *B12 deficiency* from those of B1 deficiency?	• **Vibration & position sensory loss with B12** • **No oculomotor problems with B12**
What differentiates the neurological symptoms of *vitamin E deficiency* from those of B1 deficiency?	• ***Truncal* ataxia with vitamin E** • **Psychiatric/mental status changes less prominent with vit E**
What is the name for the lower extremity problems of B12 deficiency?	**Subacute combined degeneration**
How can the name for the lower extremity problems in B12 deficiency help you remember the pathology involved?	**Subacute – comes on gradually Combined – affects both the descending pyramidal tracts (motor control) and the ascending posterior columns (sensory info)**
If untreated, what is the ultimate outcome for subacute combined degeneration of the spinal cord?	Permanent paraplegia!
Can both B12 and B1 deficiency present as psychiatric problems?	Yes
What are the hallmarks of B12 deficiency? **(4)**	1. **Megaloblastic anemia** 2. **Hypersegmented PMNs** 3. **Subacute combined degeneration of the spinal cord** 4. **Personality/psychiatric changes**
What is the other name for vitamin B12?	**Cobalamin**
Where does vitamin B12 come from?	**Synthesized by meat-related microorganisms (not found in vegetables)**
Are ovo-lacto vegetarians in danger of developing dietary B12 deficiency?	**No –** **There is plenty in eggs/milk products**
On the boards, cobalamin deficiency occurs in what patient populations, mainly? **(2 examples)**	• **Vegans (pure vegetarians)** • **Patients with pernicious anemia (intrinsic factor problems)**

What interesting physiological fact makes B12 unique among water-soluble vitamins?

It is stored for a long term in the liver!

(That's why deficiency is relatively uncommon, even among vegans)

If you wanted to look for possible B12 deficiency with a lab test, how can you do that?
(3 ways)

1. Plasma level
2. Urinary methylmalonic acid level
3. Schilling test for adequate gut absorption

How can you differentiate the neurological signs of vitamin E deficiency from those of B12?
(3)

- Pyramidal effects (weakness) with B12
- No oculobulbar with B12
- No truncal ataxia

A patient presents in high-output heart failure, with a dilated cardiomyopathy. This is one of the most serious complications of which vitamin deficiency/syndrome?

- **B1**
- **Wet beriberi**

What is the underlying cause for the high cardiac output in wet beriberi?

Peripheral vasodilation

What is "dry" beriberi?

Polyneuritis

Foot drop and wrist drop are classic presentations of which vitamin deficiency/syndrome?

- **B1**
- **Dry beriberi**

Which parts of the nervous system are affected in dry beriberi?

Peripheral motor & sensory nerves, and reflexes (usually symmetric)

Thiamine deficiency has an unusual presentation in young infants. What is it?

Aphonic beriberi – the vocal cords are partially or fully paralyzed producing a hoarse cry or no cry at all

What is the outcome of untreated thiamine deficiency in infants?

Fatal

Most infants who develop thiamine deficiency present at what age?

2–3 months
(It is usually due to low thiamine level in the breast milk)

Can infants present with neurological symptoms of thiamine deficiency?

Yes –
Includes seizures and choreiform movements when it happens in infants, though

What are the three presentations of thiamine deficiency in young infants?

1. Pseudomeningitic (neurological)
2. Wet beriberi
3. Aphonic (vocal cord paralysis)

What is the other name for vitamin C?   **Ascorbic acid**

What happens if you become vitamin C deficient?

Scurvy!
- **Swollen, bleeding gums**
- **Bruising & petechiae**
- **Anemia**
- **Poor wound healing**

What four important specific functions does vitamin C do for the body?

1. Facilitates iron absorption in the gut
2. Necessary for collagen synthesis (hydroxylation of proline & lysine)
3. Mitochondrial fatty acid supply
4. Cofactor for conversion of dopamine → norepi

Mnemonic to remember vitamin C's role in connective tissue?

Vitamin <u>C</u> <u>C</u>ross-links <u>C</u>ollagen

Which vitamins are *not* fat soluble?

B-complex & C

Supplementation of which vitamin has been found to be helpful for Ehlers–Danlos patients?

Vitamin C –
(Improves abnormal collagen hydroxylation in these patients)

What helpful function does vitamin C have for the body as a whole, along with other vitamins and molecules?

Antioxidant/free radical scavenger

Ingestion of vitamin C enhances absorption of what important metal?

Iron

If you want to confirm vitamin C deficiency with lab tests, what tests can you order?

Plasma or urinary levels

Can too much vitamin C cause a problem?

Yes –
Associated with kidney stones

Megaloblastic anemia, combined with neurological problems = which vitamin deficiency?	B12
What is the special name for the anemia that develops with B12 deficiency?	Pernicious anemia
If a child develops anemia due to B12 deficiency, what is the usual cause (in general terms)?	**Genetic disorder affecting intrinsic factor (needed for B12 absorption in the ileum)**
Which vitamin's functions are closely related to folic acid's?	B12
Why are folic acid's functions so closely related to the supply of this other vitamin?	Without B12 folic acid cannot convert to its active form
What is B12's main overall function in the body?	Synthesis of DNA
Can a B12-deficient breastfeeding Mom (e.g., a Mom who is vegan or who has pernicious anemia) pass on B12 deficiency to her infant?	**Yes**
What are the main problems associated with folic acid deficiency? (3)	1. **Macrocytic, megaloblastic anemia** 2. **Neural tube defects** 3. **Sprue-like GI symptoms (due to the enterocytes' large need for folate)**
Where is folate absorbed?	The duodenum
What biochemical marker of folate deficiency may contribute to heart disease?	↑ **Plasma homocysteine levels**
Does the USA supplement the food supply with folate?	**Yes –** **Grains have been fortified since 1998**
Deficiency of which vitamin causes "pellagra?"	**B3**

What are the three typical consequences of B3 deficiency, which all happen to start with a "D?"	**D̲iarrhea** **D̲ermatitis** **D̲ementia** (& **D̲eath**)
If you put together all of the symptoms of vitamin B3 deficiency, what are they? (Review question)	**Diarrhea, Dermatitis, Dementia, Glossitis** (For the poetry minded: Fast bowels yield diarrhea & irritation dermatitis; Thoughts slowed by Dementia, And tongue by Glossitis. Woe is me when I am low on B3!)
What is the other name for B3?	**Niacin**
Why is B3 biochemically important?	It makes NAD and NADP
Is there any downside to taking too much B3?	Flushing Vasodilation Uncomfortable
In addition to niacin, what are the other terms that can also be used to mean "vitamin B3?"	Nicotinamide Nicotinic acid
Which B vitamin can be synthesized, if sufficient quantities are not available in the diet?	Niacin (Requires tryptophan – which is an essential amino acid)
What is the classic diet for inducing B3 deficiency, and why?	Corn diet – Low in both niacin & tryptophan
What beneficial effect does niacin have, when given at pharmacological doses?	Improves lipid profile (reduces risk of atherosclerosis)
What foods contain biotin?	Most foods
Why is biotin important to the body?	It is part of four important carboxylases (two citric acid cycle enzymes, one fatty acid enzyme, and one amino acid enzyme)
How common is biotin deficiency?	Not common (rare)

How does dietary biotin deficiency present?

Dermatitis
Enteritis

What causes biotin deficiency?

Antibiotic or anticonvulsant use
(*especially with biotin-deficient total parenteral nutrition*)

&

Ingestion of *raw* eggs

(**Avidin in egg whites avidly binds biotin**)

Which type of biotin deficiency can cause muscle & nervous system problems?

Congenital biotinidase deficiency

(biotin loss is excessive, because the enzyme is needed to recycle it)

How is biotin deficiency treated?

Oral biotin

What is the fancy name for vitamin B5?

Pantothenate

Mnemonic:
Mispronounce it as "penta"thenate. Penta means "5," as in the word pentagram

Why is vitamin B5 important to the body?

It is CoA

(In our food, it is CoA. It is altered in the gut for absorption, then CoA is regenerated)

Is pantothenate deficiency common (also known as pantothenic acid)?

No –
Was seen in some WWII prisoners of war with "burning feet," though

What are the symptoms of pantothenate deficiency?

A variety of mild neuro symptoms, and vague GI complaints

(Use the "burning feet" POWs to remind you of the mild neuro system complaints)

What is the other name for vitamin B6?

Pyridoxine

**Mnemonic:
Six has an X in it like pyridoxine does!**

What does B6 deficiency cause in very young infants?

Seizures

What are the neurological consequences of vitamin B6 deficiency in older children?

Depression & confusion

Although it is more famous for causing seizures, what hematological problem can occur with B6 deficiency?

Microcytic, hypochromic anemia

Can B6 deficiency be confirmed via lab test?

Yes –
Urinary level or
Erythrocyte aminotransferase activity

Which two medications sometimes can cause vitamin B6 deficiency?

- **INH**
- **Oral contraceptives**

How is B6 deficiency treated?

Oral B6 – even if it is a genetic disorder causing the deficiency

If a patient is described as "yellow, but not jaundiced," what is the diagnosis?

Too much β-carotene (from orange foods)

How can you tell that a yellow patient is not actually jaundiced?

The sclerae & oral mucosa don't turn yellow – just the skin (in β-carotene excess)

β-carotene is a precursor form of which vitamin?

A

Mnemonic:
Because it comes from foods like carrots that are "good for your eyes/retinas" – and you know vitamin A is good for your eyes

Tocopherol is the fancy name for which vitamin?

E

Retinol or retinoic acid is the fancy name for which vitamin?

A
(like the brand name "retin-A")

What is the most common cause of early childhood blindness worldwide?

Vitamin A deficiency

Too much vitamin A is famous for causing which neurological problem?

Pseudotumor cerebri
(↑ ICP, headache, no structural abnormalities)

Too much vitamin A is famous for causing what skin problem?

Dry, cracked skin

An adolescent patient is presented with asymptomatic elevation of LFTs. Her PMH and family history are unremarkable. She has scars on her face from acne, but it appears to be well managed now. What likely culprit should you enquire about?

Isotretinoin use – it can elevate liver enzymes

What is isotretinoin's relationship to vitamins?

It is a vitamin A analog

What two important things must you check if you are considering treating a patient with isotretinoin?

Pregnancy (teratogen)

&

Liver function tests (LFTs)

What is the other name for vitamin B2?

Riboflavin

Mnemonic:
Mispronounce as ri-2-flavin
to remember it's B2

Why is B2 biochemically important?

It is the substrate that allows the body to make FMN & FAD

What problems would you expect in a patient not getting enough B2? (4)

1. **Angular cheilosis/stomatitis (sores at the lateral angle of the lips)**
2. *Keratitis/corneal neovascularization*
3. **Anemia**
4. **Tongue, skin, & neuro changes**

Which pediatric group is at unusually high risk for riboflavin deficiency?

Babies on phototherapy (B2 is very sensitive to UV radiation)

Mnemonic:
Think of the rock group the B52's giving a concert in the hot sun at a beach and losing their nutrients due to all of the effort in the hot sun

What aspect of the diet increases B2 absorption?	Fiber (more fiber, more absorption)
When B2 deficiency occurs, is it likely to occur as an isolated deficiency?	No – Multiple nutrients are usually deficient
Phytates impair the absorption of zinc. Do they have a negative impact on the absorption of other nutrients?	Yes – Iron
What makes a trace element "essential?"	**Deficiency causes problems** **(too much may also cause problems)**
"Trace" elements are usually what sort of element (on the periodic table)?	**Metals**
In times of physiological stress, levels of trace elements sometimes decrease acutely. Why?	Some are acute-phase reactants (they often redistribute out of plasma and into the liver)
Which trace element is often deficient in North American patients, who are otherwise well nourished? Why?	• Zinc • Processing food often removes the zinc content
Supplementation of trace elements sometimes causes problems when more than one is given. What is the usual underlying reason problems occur?	Usually, they compete with each other for absorption, when given PO
Why does iron deficiency increase the likelihood of a child developing lead toxicity?	**If the transporters aren't busy transporting iron, they will transport more lead than usual**
What is zinc's most important function in the body?	Transcription of DNA (by allowing transcription factors to bind to DNA)
Zinc deficiency always produces what abnormality, even when the deficiency is mild?	**Decreased growth velocity (or growth arrest)**
Does zinc supplementation correct the abnormalities seen in zinc deficiency?	**Yes**

Diarrhea is related to zinc in two important ways. What are they?

Deficiency causes diarrhea

Diarrhea significantly increases zinc losses/needs

What are the neuropsychiatric manifestations of significant zinc deficiency?

Irritability
Lethargy
Depression/anhedonia

Genetically induced zinc deficiency is called _____?

Acrodermatitis enteropathica

In general terms, what is the mechanism of genetically based zinc deficiency?

Abnormal zinc absorption by the gut

Is the clinical syndrome seen in genetically induced zinc deficiency different from what we see in patients with dietary deficiency?

No

How is acrodermatitis enteropathica inherited?

Autosomal recessive

Zinc deficiency often presents during what period of infancy?

Weaning from breast milk
(breast milk has a protein that facilitates zinc absorption)

If zinc deficiency is not treated, what is the prognosis?

Fatal – usually via infectious disease

What types of infections are zinc-deficient patients at special risk to develop?

Bacterial & monilial

(monilial = candida)

Premature & low-birth-weight infants are at special risk for zinc deficiency. Why?

- Immature transport mechanisms in the gut
- Larger losses
- Higher need due to rapid growth

How is the diagnosis of zinc deficiency made?

Clinical findings & response to supplementation –
No adequate lab or other measures have been found

What does a patient with acrodermatitis enteropathica look like?

Perioral/perianal rash & alopecia
(most obvious signs)

Is the treatment for acrodermatitis enteropathica different from the treatment for significant dietary zinc deficiency?

No –

Supplement elemental zinc (40–50 mg)

Diarrhea is known to increase zinc requirements. How big is the increase in zinc requirements with significant diarrhea?

10× increase
(even with IV zinc administration)

A patient with significant zinc deficiency is being treated with oral supplements. He or she develops a new hemolytic anemia. What is the likely cause?

Copper deficiency –

Copper and zinc are competing for transport in the gut. The unusually large amount of zinc is interfering with adequate absorption of copper

There is a famous food interaction that prevents normal absorption of zinc. What is it?

Phytates from vegetables

What is the best dietary source for zinc?

Meat
(& other animal products)

How does biotin deficiency look similar to acrodermatitis enteropathica?

Both have perioral rash & alopecia

How is biotin deficiency different from the zinc deficiency presentation of acrodermatitis enteropathica?

Biotin deficiency <u>also has ataxia</u>

What is the main purpose of copper in living organisms (including people)?

Cellular respiration
(along with iron, of course)

What are the main clinical signs of copper deficiency?

- **Nonimmune hemolytic anemia**
- **Neutropenia**
- **Osteoporosis**

What specific bone abnormalities are seen in copper deficiency?

Cupping and "sickle-shaped" spurs

Why would copper problems lead to bone problems, including osteoporosis?

Needed for collagen cross-linking

Mnemonic:
Vitamin C & Copper Cross-link Collagen!

What is the other name for Menkes kinky hair syndrome?

Menkes Steely hair syndrome (same thing)

True or False. Most circulating copper is bound to a plasma protein?

True –
90 % bound to the glycoprotein ceruloplasmin
(the rest is bound to other proteins or amino acids)

If infants are fed regular cow's milk (not formula), what metal deficiencies are they at risk for?

Copper
 &
Iron

If a patient doesn't have adequate amounts of copper in the diet, what happens to the serum copper level and the serum ceruloplasmin level?

Both low

If a patient has a hypochromic anemia that doesn't respond to iron supplementation, what other cause should you consider?

Copper deficiency

Anemia due to copper deficiency is usually accompanied by what other findings?

Neutropenia
Osteoporosis
Low serum copper
Low serum ceruloplasmin
(usually)

How is copper deficiency treated?

Oral or IV supplementation

Do term infants have a significant amount of copper stored from the fetal period the same way they have an iron store?

Yes

Do premature infants have a significant amount of copper stored prior to birth?

**Generally, no –
The storage happens shortly before birth
(same for iron)**

Do premature infants need more copper than term infants?	**Yes**
Does the body have a way to excrete excess copper?	**Yes –** **Bile secretion**
Which foods are especially known for their high copper content?	Oysters/shellfish Nuts & chocolate Liver & kidney
What household exposure can lead to copper toxicity?	Milk in brass containers (a cause of "Indian childhood cirrhosis")
What is fluoride's effect on teeth, in very general terms? **(2 effects)**	1. **Helpful – Prevents dental caries** 2. **Harmful – Too much causes fluorosis**
How does fluorosis harm the teeth?	**Undermineralization of tooth enamel making it flaky and opaque**
The protective effects of fluoride come from fluoride molecules in what part of the body?	In the saliva, itself
Is there a fluoride level at which fluorosis *won't* occur?	No
What is the most common cause of CNS damage worldwide? (Metabolic cause, not trauma)	**Iodine deficiency**
Iodine deficiency beginning at an early age causes what problem?	**Cretinism –** **Two forms: neurologic & myxedematous**
What are the typical signs of neurological cretinism? **(4)**	1. **Severe MR** 2. **Deaf & mute** 3. **Strabismus** 4. **Spastic diplegia (bilateral spasticity of legs)**
Which type of cretinism is most common?	**Neurological**

What are the typical signs of myxedematous cretinism?

Delayed DTR relaxation!!
Lack of facial expression
Sparse, coarse hair
Cool, pale skin

Also have delayed sexual development & delayed or impaired skeletal development

Children with cretinism of either type have a typical appearance. What is it?

Coarse facies with big tongue, large head size, and obvious MR by age 6 months

Is endemic goiter (iodine deficiency) common in any *developed* countries?

Yes –
Areas of Central & Western Europe

What pattern of TFTs do you expect with iodine deficiency?

The main tipoff is:
Low T4 & normal T3

If an area is just slightly low on iodine, what do you expect to see in the population living there?

Goiter, but not until adolescence or pregnancy

What is a great dietary source of iodine?

Fish

What is a great dietary source of iodine you wouldn't normally think of?

Milk –
Mainly due to the iodine compounds used on the cow's teats as antiseptic!

How is iodine deficiency corrected?

Oral or IM depot injection

What is the easiest way to evaluate for possible iodine deficiency?

Spot urine check for iodide (correlates well to recent iodine intake)

If too little iodine causes goiter, what is the effect of too much iodine?

Goiter, also!
(Can also cause thyroiditis, hyper or hypothyroidism)

Which patients are most susceptible to iodine toxicity?

Those who had chronic iodine deficiency

Chromium is primarily important for regulation of what metabolic process?

Use of glucose/cofactor for insulin

Is chromium deficiency a common problem?	No
In what two situations is chromium deficiency most often an issue?	Malnutrition & Long-term TPN
If chromium deficiency is suspected, how is it treated in malnourished children?	Single dose (of 250 μg)
When do energy requirements begin to differ between girls & boys?	**11 years**
At what age are protein requirements different for girls & boys?	**15 years**
When in life are protein requirements per kilogram of body weight greatest?	Infants (slowly declines from there)
Breastfeeding infants obtain what percentage of their calories from fat?	50 %!!!
Is it alright for a mother to breast-feed if she has an inborn metabolic error?	Sometimes – Galactosemia & tyrosinemia *not* okay
If a Mom is breast-feeding and wants to store some milk in the refrigerator, how long does she have to use it?	**5 days!**
At what temperature should refrigerated breast milk be stored?	4 °C
How long do you have to use frozen breast milk?	3–6 months
Elemental formulas are also known as _____?	Protein hydrosylates
Why are medium-chain triglycerides an important component of formula for preemies?	Decreased availability of bile acids and enzymes (MCTs don't need them)
What is the average number of meals per day eaten by adolescents?	1–2 meals per day (not good)

At about 2 years old, what percentage of the total calories should come from fat?

<30 %

What are the main reasons that enteral feeding is preferred to parenteral feeding (even if it is done via G- or J-tube)?

     (5 items including nature of nutrition & complictions)

1. More complete nutrition
2. Trophic effect on the gut
3. Lower chance of bacteremia
4. Fewer metabolic problems
5. Cheaper

Index

A
Aagenaes syndrome, 109
Abdominal adhesions, 98
Abdominal epilepsy, 18
Abdominal migraine, 18
Abdominal pain, 7, 11, 16, 18, 48, 50, 52,
    53, 55–58, 72, 78, 97, 130, 164
Abetalipoproteinemia, 103–105
Acanthocyte, 103, 105
Achalasia, 86, 128
Acholic stools, 19
Acrodermatitis enteropathica, 110, 177, 178
Adenocarcinoma, 8, 37, 78, 88
Alagille syndrome, 125
Albumin, 22, 23, 112, 129, 141, 142
Anal fissure, 130
Anorectal manometry, 46
Anorexia, 13, 53, 101, 164
Antibiotics ciprofloxacin, 9Anticholinergics,
    14, 80
Antitrypsin allele, 20
α-1-Antitrypsin deficiency, 18–20
Antral webs, 94
Antrum, 13
Anus, 5, 43, 44, 67
Appendiceal abscesses, 21
Appendiceal tumor, 6
Appendicitis, 20, 21, 55, 110, 120
Appendix, 6, 20, 21
ARDS, 57
Arthralgia, 42
5-ASA compounds, 11
Ascending cholangitis, 27
Ascites, 16, 19, 21–24, 30, 47, 59, 60
Ascorbic acid, 170
Asterixis, 131
Asthma, 57, 85, 154

Atresia, 73, 95, 97, 98
Auerbach's plexi, 5, 98
Autoimmune-related disorders, 8

B
Barrett's esophagus, 88, 89
B12 deficiency, 8, 105, 106, 168, 169, 171
Bezoars, 24, 26
Biliary atresia, 26, 27, 113
Biliary dyskinesia, 27, 28
Biliary obstruction, 114, 136
Bilirubin, 1–3, 26, 29, 113, 115, 131
    elevation, 19
    pathway, 1–2
Biotin, 172, 173, 178
Bitot spot, 138
Bloating, 17, 43, 52, 72
β-Blockers, 18, 65, 91
Blount's disease, 154
Body mass index (BMI), 134, 139, 152
Boerhaave tear, 90
Bowel rest, 8, 48, 57, 79, 120, 124
Breast feeding, 28, 29, 105, 110, 143, 182
Breast milk jaundice, 28, 29
Budd–Chiari syndrome, 63

C
Calories, 28, 87, 114, 129, 133, 140, 143, 147,
    149–151, 153, 156–158, 182, 183
Carcinoid syndrome, 6
Carcinoid tumors, 6
Caroli disease, 124, 125
Casein:whey ratio, 156
Catabolic stressor, 141
Cavernous transformation, 29

CBC, 20, 35, 139–141
Celiac disease, 30–32, 100, 101, 119
Celiac sprue, 100
Cervical esophagostomy, 76
Cholecystectomy, 28, 32
Cholecystitis, 126
Cholestasis, 19, 20, 26, 71, 109, 112
Chromium, 181, 182
Chronic active hepatitis, 10, 33, 34
Chronic constipation, 5, 38, 45
Chylomicron, 103, 105
Cirrhosis, 16, 19, 35, 59, 63, 71, 109, 117, 127
Cirrhotic ascitic fluid, 22
Cleft lip & palate, 83, 84
CNS, 40, 53, 161, 180
Coagulopathy, 15, 16, 65, 82
Cobalamin, 168
Colectomy, 10, 111
Colic, 33
Colon, 5, 9, 10, 21, 36, 38, 46, 60, 71, 77,
    80, 92
Colon cancer, 10
Colonic polyps, 83
Colonoscopy, 8, 10, 78, 121
Colostrum, 144, 155, 156
Complete rectal prolapse, 67
Congenital diarrhea, 106
Congenital hepatic fibrosis, 35, 124
Congenital microvillus disease, 106
Constipation, 5, 10, 35, 36, 38, 41, 45, 48, 53,
    68, 69, 87, 123
Copper, 107, 108, 139, 178–180
Cow's milk, 39, 139, 143, 146, 148, 149, 151,
    156, 179
Craniotabes, 161
Crigler–Najjar types 1 & 2, 114, 115
Crohn's disease, 7–9, 13, 36–38, 59, 78, 151
Crypt abscesses, 10, 78
Cryptitis, 10
CT scanning, 8
Currant jelly stools, 50
Cushing's syndrome, 152
Cyclic vomiting, 128, 129
Cyclosporine, 9, 79
Cystic fibrosis, 33, 57, 68, 69, 136, 137

D
Decreased milk production, 144
Dermatitis herpetiformis, 119, 120
Diarrhea, 6, 7, 10, 17, 18, 21, 37, 40, 43, 45,
    52, 68, 70, 72, 73, 78, 87, 100–102,
    105, 106, 109, 110, 138, 142, 146, 150,
    153, 167, 172, 177, 178
Dietary Reference Intakes (DRIs), 142

Digestive system, 5, 91
Diphtheria, 89
Distal gut, 5
Diuretics, 23
Down syndrome, 33, 95, 98, 119
DRIs. *See* Dietary Reference Intakes (DRIs)
Dry beriberi, 169
Dry skin, 138, 166
Dubin–Johnson syndrome, 115, 125
Duodenal atresia, 95
Duodenal lesions, 8
Dupuytren's contractures, 35
Dysfunction of PTEN gene, 122
Dysphagia, 39, 86, 89, 128
Dysregulation, 7

E
Ectopic mucosa, 54, 95
Ehlers–Danlos syndrome, 127, 170
Elastase, 18
Elemental diet, 8
Elemental formulas, 17, 182
Embryonic gut tissue, 6
Encopresis, 38
Endemic goiter, 181
Endoscopic retrograde cholangiopancreatography
    (ERCP), 32, 62
Endoscopy, 8, 10, 41, 86, 91, 93, 99, 100,
    127, 219
Enterochromaffin cells, 6
Enterocolitis, 5, 17, 45, 46, 60
Enterography, 8
Enteropathy, 30, 82, 102, 141
Eosinophilic gastritis, 14
Epigastric pain, 13, 99
Epi-Pen, 39
ERCP. *See* Endoscopic retrograde
    cholangiopancreatography (ERCP)
Esophageal anastomosis, 76
Esophageal atresia, 66, 74–76
Esophageal varices, 64, 91
Esophagitis, 89, 93, 127
Essential fatty acid, 137, 150

F
Failure to thrive (FTT), 5, 27, 30, 45, 73,
    104, 112
Familial adenomatous polyposis coli, 111
Fistula, 7, 9, 36, 38, 43, 44, 58, 74–76
Flatulence, 17, 43, 52, 101
Fluoride, 148, 180
Fluorosis, 148, 180
Folate, 9, 79, 101, 142, 165, 171

Folic acid, 171
Food allergy, 38–40
Foremilk, 155
Formulas, 135, 144
Foveolar cell hyperplasia, 13
FTT. *See* Failure to thrive (FTT)
Fundoplication, 77, 88

G

Gallstones, 32, 56, 69, 101
Gardner's syndrome, 121
Gastric duplication, 94, 95
Gastric outlet obstruction, 94
Gastric varices, 14
Gastric volvulus, 95, 96
Gastritis, 14, 40, 41, 73
Gastroschisis, 122, 123
GERD, 55, 77, 85–88
GE reflux, 39, 42, 150
Giardia, 13, 42, 43
Giardiasis, 43
Gilbert's syndrome, 114, 115
GI tract, 6, 53, 111
Glucose–galactose malabsorption, 102, 103
Grazing, 149
Growth failure, 8, 10, 17, 65, 137
Growth hormone deficiency, 152
Gut inflammation, 7, 52

H

H2 blockers, 14, 41, 70, 87, 88
Hemachromatosis, 51
Hematemesis, 13, 30, 66, 89
Hematochezia, 17
Henoch–Schönlein purpura (HSP), 43, 48, 126
Hepatic encephalopathy, 131
Hepatitis, 10, 19, 23, 33, 34, 81, 113, 115, 117, 118, 127, 136
Hepatitis A, 81, 115, 116
Hepatitis B, 34, 116–118
Hepatitis C, 118
Hepatitis D, 118
Hepatitis E, 118
Hepatocytes, 15, 35
Hepatofugal flow, 64
Hepatoportoenterostomy, 26, 113
Hepatorenal syndrome, 23
Hepatosplenomegaly, 19, 30, 35, 127
5-HIAA, 6
Hind, 155
Hirschsprung's disease, 5, 44–46, 97, 98
24-Hour urine, 6
H. pylori, 13, 14, 41, 99, 100, 129

HSP. *See* Henoch–Schönlein purpura (HSP)
Hydrocortisone enemas, 9
Hydrops, 126, 127
Hypercalcemia, 164
Hypermetabolic, 142
Hyperplastic, 13, 14
Hyperplastic gastropathy, 13
Hypertension, 133, 154
Hypoalbuminemia, 22
Hypocalcemia, 57, 107, 110, 137
Hypochlorhydria, 13, 25
Hypoganglionosis, 123
Hypoglycemia, 82, 131
Hypomagnesemia, 107
Hypothyroidism, 112, 152, 181

I

Ileoanal anastomosis, 79
Ileum, 32, 70, 71, 95, 105, 171
Imerslund syndrome, 105
Immunoglobulins, 155
Immunosuppressives, 34, 38, 79
Immunosuppressives azathioprine, 9
Imperforate anus, 43, 44
Incontinence, 5, 38
Inflammatory bowel disease, 7, 34
Infliximab, 9
Inguinal hernias, 46
Inguinal lymphadenopathy, 48
Intestinal neuronal dysplasia, 123
Intestinal obstruction, 45, 48, 49
Intestinal volvulus, 82
Intussusception, 43, 48–51, 54, 55, 68, 111, 130
Intussusception presentation, 50
Intussusceptions, 43, 48–51, 54, 55, 68, 111, 130
Iodine, 180, 181
Iron, 8, 37, 51, 71, 78, 89, 101, 109, 129, 135, 136, 147, 150, 151, 157, 165, 170, 176, 178, 179
Iron ingestion, 51, 52
Irritable bowel syndrome, 52

J

Jaundice, 16, 19, 25, 28, 29, 95, 126
Jejunum, 42, 71
Johanson–Blizzard syndrome, 112
Juvenile polyposis, 120, 121
Juvenile polyps, 120

K

Kasai, 26, 113, 125
Kawasaki disease, 126

Kayser–Fleischer ring, 108
Kidney stones, 69, 78, 164, 171
Kwashiorkor, 129, 140, 158, 159

L
Lactase, 11, 12, 53
Lactase deficiency, 11–12, 53, 72, 119, 146
Lactose, 12, 53, 102, 119, 146, 156
    intolerance, 17, 18, 42, 52, 53
    malabsorption, 12
"Ladd" procedure, 82
LeVeen shunts, 24
Liver, 2, 3, 6, 15, 16, 18–20, 22–24, 26, 27, 30,
    34, 35, 59, 60, 63–66, 71, 81, 82, 97,
    107–109, 112–115, 117, 125–127, 129,
    131, 136, 159, 163, 169, 175, 176, 180
Lymphoma, 8, 14, 31, 100, 121
Lymphopenia, 140

M
Macrocytic anemia, 123
Magnesium deficiency, 137
Magnetic resonance (MR), 8, 180, 181
Mallory–Weiss tear, 91
Malnutrition, 68, 129, 134, 140–141,
    158, 182
Malrotation, 66, 82, 95–98, 129
MALT lymphoma, 100
Marasmus, 129, 140, 158, 159
Marfan syndrome, 127
McBurney's point, 20
Meckel's diverticulum, 53, 54
Meconium ileus, 96–98
Meissner effect, 5, 98
Menetrier disease, 129
Menkes kinky hair syndrome, 107, 179
Menkes syndrome, 107
6-Mercaptopurine, 9, 11, 79
Mesenteric adenitis, 54, 55
Metronidazole, 9, 11, 43, 100
Microcytic anemia, 31
Migraine headaches, 18
Milk allergy, 17, 55, 56
Mother's milk, 55, 144, 155, 156
MR. See Magnetic resonance (MR)
Murphy's sign, 32
Myxedematous cretinism, 181

N
Necrotizing enterocolitis, 60
Neonatal hemochromatosis, 109

Neonatal jaundice, 19, 26
Neonatal period, 5, 44, 45
Neoplasm, 14
Nesidioblastosis, 112
Neural crest cells, 5, 6
Neurological cretinism, 180
Neuropathy, 34, 103
Neutraceutical, 142
Niacin, 166, 172
Night blindness, 166
Nipple pain, 145
Nodular regenerative hyperplasia, 16
Noncirrhotic portal hypertension, 16
Nonfamilial hyperinsulinemic
    hypoglycemia, 112
Non-IgE mediated, 17
NSAIDs, 10, 18, 30, 99, 127
Nutrition, 8, 27, 40, 133–183

O
Obesity, 139, 151–154, 157
Obstruction, 2, 6, 7, 15, 22, 24, 26, 27, 29, 30,
    35, 36, 38, 45, 48, 49, 51, 54, 56, 62,
    64, 66, 72, 82, 83, 85, 94, 97, 98, 111,
    114, 136
Oculobulbar muscle dysfunction, 137
Odynophagia, 86, 130
Omphalocele, 122, 123
Ophthalmoplegia, 137
Osteomalacia, 160
Ostomy, 151
Overdistended, 5
Overweight, 134, 152

P
Palmar erythema, 34, 35
pANCA, 78
Pancolitis, 80
Pancreatectomy, 112
Pancreatic exocrine dysfunction, 123
Pancreatic pseudocyst, 61, 62
Pancreatitis, 23, 25, 32, 56–58, 62, 109, 111,
    112, 123, 124
Pantothenate, 173
Paralytic ileus, 48
Paraplegia, 168
Parenteral nutrition, 8, 70, 71, 107, 173
Parenteral nutrition liver disease (PNLD), 71
Pearson syndrome, 123
Pellagra, 166, 167, 171
Pentasa, 9
Peptic ulcer disease, 99, 100, 130

Peptides, 6
Perianal disease, 7
Perianal rashes, 69
Perirectal abscess, 58, 59
Peutz–Jegher, 48, 111
PFIC. *See* Progressive familial intrahepatic
    cholestasis (PFIC)
Phylloquinone, 163
Phytates, 135, 176, 178
Phytobezoar, 25
Pigeon chest, 160
Pleural effusion, 57, 91
Plummer–Vinson syndrome, 89
Pneumatosis intestinalis, 50, 61
PNLD. *See* Parenteral nutrition liver disease
    (PNLD)
Polyarteritis nodosa, 116
Polyhydramnios, 74, 75, 94, 105
Polyneuritis, 169
Portal hypertension, 16, 20, 24, 27, 35, 63–66,
    71, 124
Post-cholecystectomy syndrome, 27
Prader–Willi syndrome, 27
Prealbumin, 141, 142
Prednisone, 9, 11
Primary malnutrition, 140
Processus vaginalis, 47
Proctitis, 11, 68
Progressive familial intrahepatic cholestasis
    (PFIC), 109
PROlactin, 144
Protein-energy malnutrition, 140, 141
Protein-losing enteropathy, 82, 102, 141
Protein-losing gastropathy, 13, 129
Proteus syndrome, 121, 122
Proton pump inhibitor, 85–88
Proximal, 5, 10, 42, 44, 54, 72, 74, 89
Pseudo-Hirschsprung's disease, 123
Pseudopolyps, 10
Pseudotumor cerebri (↑ ICP, headache, no
    structural abnormalities), 175
Psoriasis, 160
Ptosis, 137
Pulmonary hypertension, 154
Purpuric skin lesions, 138
Pyloric atresia, 94
Pyloric stenosis, 66, 67, 93
Pyridoxine, 173

R
Rachitic rosary, 136, 160, 162
Ramstedt procedure, 67
Recommended Daily Allowance, 142

Rectal/anal tone, 5
Rectal ulcers, 68
Reference Daily Intake & Daily Reference
    Values, 143
Reflux, 41, 42, 57, 70, 75, 77, 84, 85, 87–89,
    150, 151
Regenerating mucosa, 10
Retention, 105
Retinitis pigmentosa, 104, 105
Retinoic acid, 174
Retinol, 138, 166, 174
Retrocecal appendix, 21
Reye's syndrome, 81, 82
Rib flaring, 162
Riboflavin, 175
Richter hernia, 48
Rickets, 34, 107, 110, 136, 147, 159–163
Rowasa, 9

S
Salivary gland tumor, 83
Salivary hemangiomas, 83
Salivary lymphangiomas, 83
SBP. *See* Spontaneous bacterial peritonitis
    (SBP)
Sclerosing cholangitis, 8, 10, 34, 78
Sclerotherapy, 64, 65, 83
Scrotal raphe, 44
Scurvy, 170
Secondary malnutrition, 140
Sengstaken–Blakemore tube, 65
Sepsis, 24, 29, 42, 45, 59, 60, 80
Serotonin metabolites, 6
Short bowel syndrome, 69, 70, 101
Shwachman–Diamond syndrome, 111, 112
Sickle cell, 32
Sigmoid volvulus, 36
Single mediastinal tumor, 23
Skin
    folds, 139
    lesion, 8, 36, 37, 77
Sleep apnea, 154
Small bowel, 6, 8, 31, 69–71, 101, 102, 107, 130
Solid foods, 148, 157, 158
Sphincter of Oddi dysfunction, 27
Sphincterotomy, 28
Spider angiomata, 34
Splenic precaution, 30
Spontaneous bacterial peritonitis (SBP),
    22, 59, 60
Stadiometer, 140
Steatorrhea, 30, 104, 110
String sign, 66

Stunted, 134
Subacute combined degeneration, 168
Submucosa, 6, 100
Sucrase-isomaltase deficiency, 119
Sulfasalazine, 8, 9, 11, 79, 126
Superior mesenteric artery syndrome, 72
Suprahepatic, 63

T
TB peritonitis, 23
Telescoping, 49
Terminal ileum, 8, 36, 37, 60, 97
Thiamine, 167, 169, 170
Tocopherol, 166, 174
Toddler's diarrhea, 72, 73
Toxic megacolon, 5, 10, 46, 80
TPN, 11, 32, 71, 126, 139, 182
Tracheoesophageal fistul (TEF), 44, 73–77
Transilluminate a scrotal hernia, 47
Trendelenburg, 47
Triangular cord, 113
Trichobezoar, 24, 25
Trichophagia, 25
Trichotillomania, 25
Trousseau's sign, 137
Tumor, 6, 23, 37, 48, 57, 83, 100, 121
Typhlitis, 120

U
Ulcerative colitis (UC), 7, 9–10, 77–80
Umbilical hernia, 123
Upper intake (UI) level, 143
Ursodeoxycholic acid, 20
Urticaria, 42, 150

V
Variceal bleeding, 64, 65
Varix formation, 20

Vasoactive, 6
Vegetarians, 129, 143, 158, 168
Veno-occlusive liver disease, 15–16
Venous outflow obstruction, 35
Video capsule endoscopy, 8
Vitamin(s), 26, 27, 34, 37, 71, 102–104, 110,
        129, 133–183
Vitamin A, 16, 63, 138, 139, 142, 166,
        174, 175
Vitamin B1, 167–169
Vitamin B2, 175
Vitamin B5, 173
Vitamin B6, 173, 174
Vitamin B12, 8, 37, 71, 101, 105, 106, 129,
        143, 167–169, 171
Vitamin C, 129, 166, 170, 171, 179
Vitamin D, 101, 129, 136, 137, 143, 147,
        159–164
Vitamin E deficiency, 104, 137, 165, 166,
        168, 169
Volvulus, 36, 48, 82, 83, 95, 96, 98

W
Wasted, 31, 134
Weight maintenance, 153
Wernicke–Korsakoff syndrome, 167
Wet beriberi, 169, 170
Whipple disease, 120
Wilson disease, 63, 107, 108

X
Xanthomas, 27

Z
Zinc, 71, 110, 129, 135, 142,
        176–178
Zinc malabsorption, 110
Zollinger–Ellison syndrome, 13, 14, 99, 100

77825827R00117

Made in the USA
Lexington, KY
02 January 2018